Raw Feeding,
A SARF Diet
&
The key to health vitality and life longevity

Feeding By The Laws Of Nature

GW00492634

By
Alpha Canine Health

Table of Contents

Dedication

Firstly I would like to dedicate this book to all the Genuine Men and Women that have dedicated their lives to helping bring alongside sustain true health to dogs as well as Humans and other animals in general; some are with us today, many others are not, thank you, your work has assisted me on my journey along with many others by bringing real health as well as true awareness of what real nutrition is, in addition to the inner standing of the body, what creates disease and how to assist the body in healing itself.

Dr Ronald Schultz, Dr Jeannie Thomason, Dr Robert Morse, Dr Patricia Jordan, Dr Edward.E. Shook, David.L.Mech, Billinghurst, Robert.K.Wayne, Lonsdale, Brown & Taylor, Pottinger, Professor Arnold Ehret, Hippocrates, any others that I'm sure I will have missed finally Dr Sebi who assisted by helping to bring simplicity, connection, common sense and total awareness of it all.

Acknowledgments

Firstly I would like to thank God, God being the creation of all life and the energetic healing force within the body, also manifested into many forms including the natural herbs found growing abundantly in nature of which I use to assist the body through assimilation, in its unique healing process and ability. I acknowledge the importance and beauty of life, creation and am grateful to have been guided and given enlightenment that helps to bring health, vitality, and life longevity. My heart felt gratitude also goes out to the people that have seen the truth in what I speak that has given them the faith and patience resulting in their dogs and many others being given a new lease of life that is abundant in the true riches of life, which are in fact - health, vitality, and longevity.

I am forever thankful for the unconditional love and support I have been shown from the family and friends who have believed in me and supported me, you will never know how Grateful I am to have you in my life and by my side, you are all loved and appreciated very much, I thank you.

About the Author

Gareth is dedicated to everything He's passionate about; essentially, He has realised that His biggest passion is life and that true wealth is health. He seeks to find the truth that can be proven with evidence, and can be explained from application; he isn't interested in theory as such, as he believes, this comes from his engineering background as a CI engineer (Continuous Improvement engineer) and from having to find the root cause of problems. One of His gifts, as he sees, is being able to simplify information being able to put it into context using the law of association, helping most people to understand what's been taught. He has, in fact, been advised to host workshops teaching people. Gareth has dedicated much of his time to learning about dogs as a species and their nutritional requirements, this has naturally progressed into health and awareness of the body resulting in the inner standing and cause of disease. His purpose is to re-educate people, like many others have done over the course of history, with the knowledge that they are missing and essentially give people the gift of causation to disease, so that they could prevent it, which of course, leads to the cure. Gareth, however, acknowledges that there is nothing new under the sun and that the body is a self-healing mechanism proven in many ways. He would also like to point out that although some of the above might seem egotistical, his main aim is to help others, mainly because when he needed help, it simply wasn't in the system, because much of what we need for true healing is hidden. Hence in the book, he talks about treating the root cause as opposed to symptomatic.

Author's Note

When we read the books written by these beautiful souls or see videos online that are not part of the mainstream media or education systems; we can gain a different perspective on the human body and disease, its definition, and its origin. These resources hidden in the sense they aren't promoted via the mainstream channels such as television, news, papers, radio, and of course, the education system, which seems to have in many areas (where it counts) function as an indoctrination system *"the process of teaching a person or group to accept a set of beliefs uncritically."* We also find that throughout time; there have been many people aware of what we should and need to be teaching in this field rather than what's actually being taught and promoted as health in this mainstream machine, which is creating the very thing we are seeking to prevent. However, today the number of people seeing through the deception is growing and growing quicker than ever before. I am seeing a growing number of people that have an open mind, who are searching for answers (truth) and, for the first time in a long time, beginning to question what is clearly now at the tipping point where it's becoming increasingly more obvious that many approaches being taught and applied for the disease are not working. This realisation brings to light that not only are the approaches not working, but they are also, in many cases, causing most diseases, disease created by masking the root cause from treating symptoms and in fact shutting down the body's innate healing ability; in fact, it's so obvious, most Vets actually admit that they treat symptomatic! Hence there is more sickness with dogs, cats and other animals including people today than ever before. The problem is that what is happening today has been introduced gradually over time, not only this, but people are now born into a system where disease and illness are seen as natural and normal; they are born into a system that they don't even realise they need to question! However, because of greed and the fact of disease along with the current reaction and approach within the mainstream system and society, more people are seeing these issues and beginning to question their approaches and even knowledge. This is driving the search for other approaches and truth is starting to reach the masses, we are in a time where health is declining at such an alarming rate. It is in the awareness of this, together with enlightenment, that is, as I see, allowing us to see this atrocity. My aim is to help you understand this on a deeper level, essentially giving you the cure for the disease in the form of prevention.

I have had the privilege of discovering as well as reading many books over the past 10 years (old and new) as well as watching videos, realising that people have been trying to raise awareness of real health care and what that entails as well as our understanding of nutrition for 100's of years! So this book is dedicated to the souls that have fought and are fighting for truth, helping to bring back health besides vitality, which in turn is what provides life longevity; what we consume becomes us, "we are what we eat." This not only applies to Humans but to all living animals. The simple fact of the matter is, however, that this known but misunderstood phrase not only applies to what is consumed in the sense of food but also what is observed daily (IE, the environment of any animal), including the thoughts created from the environment that then trigger emotions! All that is consumed will lead to one of 2 outcomes – health, vitality, and life longevity or disease which leads to a reduced life span. Thus, the phrase I use is **'we are what we consume.'**

What we are aiming for and should achieve is health & vitality that naturally creates life longevity. I'm hoping this book will help shed some light for you, assisting you by realising how this is achieved with your dogs and with all walks of life.

What we consume becomes us – **"We are what we consume."**

This book is mainly focused on the declining health in dogs, but it will also show that the inner standing (to know at a soul level), together with the approach, is required for all species – life forms and living organisms and is applied as well as used the same on a biological level.

So with this initial introduction to 'we are what we consume,' I will proceed to identify these areas of consumption from 2 sides, matter and energy. Matter in the form of anything in a physical form as well as energy in the form of thoughts and emotions- emotions = energy in

3

motion. The aim is to show you how important our inner standings of these are to achieve health in all walks of life.

We will begin with matter and, in particular, food which should always be in the form of a SARF diet (Species Appropriate Raw Food); this is specific to the species in mind and will not only provide a substance that the body recognises thus is naturally able to process. But after the body has broken down its SARF diet, we will achieve cell assimilation, providing cell food.

The natural waste can then be eliminated efficiently to maintain homeostasis (this is how we strengthen the body at the cellular level).

Frankly put! Anything consumed (in the form of matter) that isn't part of the SARF diet either isn't recognised, so it cannot be assimilated efficiently, which means that it won't bring the strength to the cell that it should! or its acid-forming, which means that it actually breaks the cells down effecting the mucus membrane, the waste produced after processing can then be very difficult for the body to remove by elimination through the lymphatic system (body's sewer system), or we lose the ease of function from the cell. We often get this combined; this causes constipation throughout the system, which leads to inflammation – (acidosis), causing cellular degeneration. Thus, we create dis-ease within the body due to which the body is no longer able to function or operate with ease, resulting in dis-ease!

Equally, the environment in which the animal is subject to affects their emotions. Emotions are found in 2 categories positive besides negative, and are, in fact, energies! Positive or rather positivity is where we find Love, Happiness, peace, calmness, a sense of freedom, Joy, etc; these all help to create a healthy body. Whereas negative emotions (negativity) such as stress, anxiety, fear, sadness, captivity, depression, etc., all lead to dis-ease. One can say, and in fact, it is said, that love is a creative energy, which implies that everything is created from love, one could then say that destruction comes from negative energies.

Now if you're wondering how emotions affect health, it's in the understanding of chemistry and, fundamentally, energy! For example, Happiness alongside Love triggers the adrenal along with the pineal gland to secrete dopamine as well as serotonin; we will also see the hypothalamus gland release oxytocin. These 3 Hormones (hormones are chemical messengers that help cells communicate, triggering various actions within the body), assisting the body in several positive ways between them by helping to maintain calmness, movement, and motivation along with strengthening the immune system, thus creating homeostasis as well as coherence at an energetic level.

Stress or fear will trigger the adrenal glands (which sit on top of the kidneys) to release cortisol, a kind of acid. This hormone allows an animal that's under threat to enter the process of fight or flight; it can be lifesaving, allowing a deer, for example, to escape from harm even though it may have an injury or weakness (the chemistry in the body is altered and homeostasis is lost for a period of time); however, it is destructive to the body. Furthermore, when a state of stress or fear is seen continuously, it will have a negative impact on the physical body. High cortisol levels have been seen to impact the body in many ways, promoting a loss of minerals from the body and further increasing the acid load. The body can only assimilate minerals as well as other nutrients properly when the acid/alkaline PH levels are balanced, or what some will recognise as the body in homeostasis.

Under acidic conditions, enzymatic processes may be hindered, and waste products/toxins can and do become trapped in the lymphatic system (bodies sewer system); this stagnation or rather constipation is what leads to cell dysfunction from inflammation due to the waste backing up into the cell. We will also cover this in a little more detail further in the book when we identify the body as being electrical.

This book is aimed at the declining health in dogs, fixing your attention on the SARF diet rather than what's come to be known as a Raw diet, mainly due to the simple fact that all animals on earth eat a raw diet, the key. However, it is in fact, specific to the species and has to be in order to achieve its purpose. This basic understanding is and has been lost in the raw feeding sector; in addition to focusing on the SARF diet, I will also identify the effects of what's consumed as a substance being a direct link to the causation of disease, but it will also show that the inner standing along with the correct approach taken to achieve health or assist the body in regenerating itself is required for all species – life forms, living organisms thus is applied the same.

Foreword

My intention for this book is to reach out to as many people with dogs as I can, but I would also like to reach the raw feeders in general who have been given information from others that are in positions of trust, leading the public into the assumption that their dogs are omnivores. We are going to use nature (the best scientific lab we have), biology, in addition to common sense to hopefully assist you in truly understanding exactly what your dog, as a carnivore, should be consuming along with why and how disease forms, my hope is that I can also raise awareness to help bring to light that this also applies to all life forms!

As you may find from the book and as many sure4pets customers will be aware, I like to explain things in as much detail as I can but at the same time simplify the knowledge so that people can picture information in order to fully understand. Alongside this, I use the law of association to help embed the information which I base on truth from in the fieldwork or cause and effect.

I also believe that the truth is simple, much like nature itself. Furthermore simplifying (making complex things easy to understand, work with and use) was the skill that was drilled into me as a CI (continuous Improvement engineer). which actually gives us a great place to start the book. With an 'I'll try and keep it brief' introduction to my background that will hopefully paint a picture of where it started for me;

how it's helped me along the way and why I have been able to use as well as apply the same tools and knowledge provided in understanding health and is a good a place to start as any. One thing that people won't know and may not see in the shop or observe from the book is that I tend to apply myself to everything I do, giving 100% of what I have. Other than this, I always work on giving my best, particularly when theory not only makes sense, but when the evidence is present during the application of the theory, and results are visible. This can sometimes initially involve self-pressurising to understand and apply new information in order to achieve the best results, so I can best deliver this right information with passion and love (my driving force and energy), which is what I believe comes naturally with truth as energy, (which resonates at a certain frequency, by resonates I mean like when you hear someone singing and the hairs on the back of your neck stand to attention, or like we see with 2 identical tuning forks), for me the truth is what this is all about!.

Chapter 1: Where it all began for me.

I was living a normal life back in the early 2000s. I was a CI Engineer (continuous Improvement engineer) for a major <u>car parts</u> manufacturing company; my role required many skills (all provided in-house, on the job or another way to put it 'in the field') which came together to make up the TPS system (Toyota Production System). These attributes provided me the ability to improve costing, quality along with the delivery of production lines by studying them at a basic level applying tools like takt time, 2s1y, process flow, abnormality management - driven by the use of visualisation, where myself and team members or colleagues would then have to potentially design along with engineer the process (ironically what was also termed as a cell). Looking at the process flow from start to finish whilst being conscious of what added value, what was necessary or what, in fact, wasn't needed at all), this would then be followed by the engineering of workstations, measuring gauges etc. We were also often tasked with finding the root cause of a problem that existed within an existing production cell thus having an understanding of the process flow was essential. Our task also included identifying the issues at the root in order to remove and prevent them with the particular tools we were provided with. In some circumstances, this would involve going back to basics and stripping parts of the cell or the whole cell out in order to eliminate the issue, then building the cell back up from scratch! This generally happened when the line manager, supervisor or team leader had so many issues within the cell due to them bodging a job allowing them to meet the shipping requirement, which was simply suppressing and hiding the problem! ultimately, they would often end up in a position where they couldn't see the woods for the trees and ended up firefighting numerous issues.

As the company's ethos and part of the TPS system is 'just in time', production was based on what was needed for the day, having no real reserve of parts to fall back on should an issue arise. It would've been fine in a world with no issues, but should a problem appear, the risk then of a potential for missed delivery was increased. Considering the frequency of problems, this increase in the risk meant that not only were the team leaders constantly chasing shipments if any issues arose, they would, as it was termed, 'end up putting a plaster over the issue' and as mentioned would bodge the problem to then continue providing parts, essentially they were addressing the symptoms, the problem with this, is when another issue came along, they were still firefighting the first issue. In many cases, all the team leader or supervisor would do is react to problems within the cell constantly firefighting; this was simply because they hadn't dealt with the first issue at the root, suppressing the actual problem, which is exactly how we react to disease and the symptoms of disease today!

Take a mental note of this part of the book, talking about cells firefighting and rebuilding, as this is also relevant to what has assisted in my awareness as well as realisation of what is actually happening today with regards to health and the body and is the very reason, I have mentioned it; I am hoping you will see this as you get deeper into the book).

Welcome Oli

So where this journey really started for me was when my previous fiancée and I picked up our first dog Oli. My Fiancée had been on at me for some time about getting a dog. Since she had grown up with a dog, she felt it would be a good addition to our home. I, on the other hand, felt that a dog would tie us down. Besides, if I'm being truthful (which is what this is all about), I was scared of dogs; my childhood was full of bad experiences with dogs, so I wasn't all that struck by them, but after several years I finally agreed, and we began looking for what turned out to be our fur baby Oli.

Oli was, at the time, a 10-week-old British Bulldog, and I fell in love with him immediately. I saw this life that required my/our love as well as our care to thrive and ultimately live a healthy, happy life. The Breeder we picked Oli up from bred Bulldogs specifically, she had been breeding them for around 28 years. She told us that she didn't flea, worm or vaccinate any of her own dogs alongside this, she fed them with a raw diet that consisted of meat, bone and offal. I can remember her claiming that all her dogs were reaching very good life spans of between 17 to 20 years old, and she only bread healthy dogs. However, at this time and although the information had gone in, I didn't actually accept or appreciate what she had told us (like the majority of people, I was brainwashed) – As I hear it, brainwashed seems to be the wrong word, it implies cleaning, a better term I think and have already mentioned would be indoctrinated, because of the indoctrination within the system we live, I couldn't really think for myself or consciously accept that there could be an alternative or in fact, a better approach to what was being pushed, recommended as well as advised by 'professionals.' Thus, because of this, after picking Oli up and being given a week's worth of raw food from the breeder and, at the time, having very little awareness of Oli's needs, we began feeding biscuit 'food'.

When I recall, I said to My Fiancée as we got in the car after picking Oli up, 'We can't just give him raw meat; I know what the breeder has just said, but surely he needs more than just this minced raw food to live healthy' – how wrong was I!?

From picking Oli up, we finished his week of raw food the breeder had given us, which he wolved down! literally eating it within seconds. Once Oli had finished his raw we went to buy what we thought and was known to be the best dried-biscuit/kibble food costing around £75.00 for the largest bag.

We began what we thought was the start of a healthy life for Oli; however, Oli had other plans. The first time we fed Oli with biscuit, although he finished it quickly, it wasn't maintained. In fact, the following day was a different story. Since the second day, Oli had been as I saw at the time (the trap most people fall into), very fussy. He simply wouldn't entertain the biscuit anymore. He wasn't eating, so it raised concern as we really didn't know at the time what we were doing. Over a period of around 4-5 months, maybe a little longer, we tried a varying number of different brands, but Oli showed interest to none and refused to eat them. His refusal to eat the biscuit ended up with us buying whole raw chickens. At this time, due to lack of awareness feeding it to Oli cooked, which we were adding to his biscuit but didn't help at all as Oli would simply spit out any biscuit focusing on the cooked chicken along with any jelly that was in his bowl. Other than having issues with getting Oli to eat, training him had been a breeze!

At this time, I was working lots of overtime - 10 hrs a day, 7 days a week, so I didn't have much time or energy to focus on getting to the root of why Oli wouldn't eat, but I knew we were missing something, and that I had to sort it out, I had a gut-feeling that something wasn't right. Ironically, it was around this time that the overtime fell back, so I was able to start digging into why Oli was being (as we saw at the time) so fussy, thus, my Mission started. Little did I know at this time the journey I would be taking or where it would lead me to; it was to be the starting point to where I am today, helping people heal their dogs along with writing this book.

I began researching with the questions, why won't my dog eat? What's the best food for my dog, and at almost every turn, I ended up with the same answer A RAW FOOD DIET. This took me back to what the breeder had told us, moreover, it is what Oli had started his life consuming.

I have to say it took me several weeks to convince my fiancée that we should have another go with this raw diet, but once we were in agreement, we set out to source a supplier, which at this time wasn't as easy as it is today, we managed to source a local supplier to us, and we picked up Oli's raw food, the first meal we put down for Oli never touched the sides just as Oli had started his life with us loving food, wolfing it down eagerly without hesitation. At this point, my thoughts were, 'if anyone knows what he should be eating, it's Oli' it was clear this was the right food for Oli. He absolutely loved it and still does almost 10 years on!

With the weeks passing, we slowly introduced other meats finding that Oli seemed to be again becoming fussy with certain types. He had his favourites and wouldn't really entertain light meats, chicken, turkey, fish, Pheasant or duck. He wanted Beef, Lamb, & Heart or Pork, so we had to add the light meats to the red meats to get variation into him. This idea worked in a way as he was eating so much better than

15

before, so we decided to go along with it, however I was later to discover just why Oli was being fussy and this will be covered later in the book.

From this point on, I did little bits of reading/research, enough to get us by, and Oli was eating more or less every meal again. Furthermore, he was clealry enjoying his food. Welcome Charlie.

Around a year into having Oli, I decided it had gone so well with Oli, it would be good to add to the family by giving Oli a companion too. This time, it was my Fiancée that wasn't too set on bringing another dog into our home, but after much ear chewing from myself, she agreed with a condition. She gave me what I imagined was an impossible task, she said 'if you can find a white Bulldog with a brown ear, the answer is yes' after around 2 months of searching, I found Charlie surprising her with him.

Charlie was nothing like Oli, and although he settled in lovely with Oli accepting him, Charlie initially was a little terror (lol).

After getting Charlie, who had ended up as the runt of the litter (but boy, was he boisterous), we went through the same process as with Oli, microchipped with a vet check. However, although Charlie had come to us fully vet checked with no underlying issues, our Vet had picked up on a heart murmur. Charlie had a number of tests confirming that He had a stage 4 heart murmur out of 6 stages, however for as long as Charlie was with us, it never interfered with his life or general day-to-day activities, although it was always in the back of our minds, which really ended up with Charlie altering most of our house rules.

Introducing Charlie to Raw was a little different to Oli, Charlie had been weaned onto a well-known brand of biscuit that wasn't a very good quality product from what I had found out from my initial research with Oli. Upon introducing Charlie to raw, we found that all he wanted to eat was the lighter meats, Chicken, Turkey and sometimes Duck; Charlie was the total opposite of Oli, but always ate with enthusiasm along with eagerness, in fact, he would eat his own as quick as he could to get to Oli's bowl.

Time passed as it does, and through the research as well as general observations along with some trial and error (in the field experience), we had managed to get Oli together with Charlie eating a varied as well as balanced raw food diet, so things were going pretty well.

My research had picked up some pace now and I realised that the Breeder had been right about raw feeding. But I began to question why and how she could have had her dogs living to between 17 -20 years old without the need for flea, worm or vaccination treatments. Most of my research at this time took me to the US, which seemed to be about 10 years ahead of us, with regards to raw feeding along with their natural approach to health. My question at the time was 'are these treatments that we are pushed truly necessary?' We are informed they are necessary to achieve health along with vitality (with no mention of life longevity), yet we now have such a demand for pet health care? This process just didn't make any sense; something in my gut was now telling me to dig deeper into this too.

I came across many people and their research at this time, Dr Jeannie Thomason together with Dr Ronald Schultz, the Pottinger Study and others already mentioned who were very enlightening and thus helped enormously in my awareness of dogs; alongside the natural approach that helped to achieve as well as maintain health! I also came across several journalists whose names slipped my mind; due to the amount of information I was processing. However, they also presented some very interesting information and aided in doing what they set out to do, which is to create awareness and for that, I am grateful. One article I read at that time has always stuck with me; it was written by a lady that applied common sense (something we seem to have lost but comes naturally - I believe with the process of asking questions with an open mind). The journalist pointed out some interesting facts that really resonated with me and has done with thousands of people I have already spoken to. She pointed out that there are around 1 million species, billions of animals that live naturally on Earth; they all consume a raw food diet (the key being that they are specific to their species, which I will come back to later in the book), they don't have the same constant treatments - flea, worm or vaccinations and ironically there are none of the diseases in nature as we see in domesticated animals or in people. It was this that really initiated my interest further into just why disease exists and where it originates. The main lesson I saw here was that nature is where we need to be looking; as I always say – *'Nature is the best scientific lab we have!'*

With the increasing awareness and lots of reading, things became to make more sense. At the same time things at work were not so good, so I wasn't too happy. I had numerous conversations with my fiancée about what I could do; I looked at several other companies that suited my job role. However, I wanted something where the effort I put in could be reflected in the reward I received, which at the time was pay.

I decided the best thing for myself was to be self-employed. Initially, I wanted something that required a lesser number of hours. I had gone over what industry I could go into, which would be the easiest to set up, and because I could see a definite advantage to raw feeding that brought truth as well as results in the information I had gained and used, I thought the best step and most logical was a raw feeding pet shop, again little that I knew where it would lead me.

I left my job and set the ball rolling with the setup of what turned out to be sure4pets, in my mind's eye, I saw sure4pets as a natural, eco-friendly shop, with a focus on promoting pet health and vitality at its foundation. One of the many things I learnt whilst being employed was when anything new is being introduced to a production cell; generally, the operator wouldn't accept the new design; I often used to think to myself, 'What is it with people that don't like change, why are we so fixed on routine, other than with technology, new phones are accepted a new car, anything really that's to do with technology we openly and in fact blindly accept without question' then I realised that in most cases, we assume that we're getting something better, I realised that in most cases people are presented with a benefit.

I started applying the approach of showing the benefits to production operators finding that in many cases, they then accepted the new cell design. Thus, we had more success with improving production in general as the new standards were accepted, whether it made working easier or improved cost or quality of the process or product.

With the setup and opening of the shop and although I had seen the response from my boys and how well they were doing, I knew I needed to share the real benefits of feeding raw by showing others what I had discovered so far - in order to get people to realise that although we had been doing something that was the norm and had become a precedent, it wasn't right or as I had come to discover in line with nature. I also needed to inner stand the dog more as a species so I could better explain just why a SARF diet (not simply a raw diet) was not only essential, but a key part in achieving health, vitality thus naturally providing life longevity. I had to gather facts from studies that helped to prove the health benefits alongside real-life transformations that have clearly been seen. So, the addiction to research, essentially to investigation began, trial and error, using the skills I had been given as a CI engineer. These skills allowed me to observe as well as learn in the field (hands on) more about the dog as a species alongside some of their traits. More common sense was achieved thus began the process of re-educating myself along with other people, helping them to see that what they had been programmed into believing and, in most cases, blindly accepting was the wrong approach. By this I mean things become the norm, a precedent is set where people's thoughts, opinions, and questions are along the lines of - **"My Parents and Grandparents fed biscuits for years, or my previous dogs were flea'd and wormed and had vaccinations" (following the same patterns) "so how could it be wrong, or why would it be wrong, this system has been used for 100 years or so, so it must be the right?!".** But what we couldn't see (as it has been happening slowly over time) was the increase in the need for constant treatments that have ultimately led to a huge reduction in the average age and life spans of dogs (and cats) as well as an influx of veterinary practices, (proving that the above isn't working. Furthermore, it is making things worse as lifespans are getting shorter). Changing this mindset can be challenging, and getting people to see outside of the box can be hard, so at this time, I knew and still do that I, like all the others past as well as present, have our work cut out, but I do believe progress is being made, I am seeing it with my own eyes.

Chapter 2: Questioning the current paradigm.

So, now that we have established that we need to question the current paradigm, what we need to realise as part of questioning in order to change for the better, is that, in most cases, the wrong questions are asked. Mainly because people can't see other factors or the bigger picture, so people happily question change but not what they have become accustomed to doing because they didn't have the full picture. I read a few years ago that around one and a half century ago, dogs lived up to 20. They were fed mainly butchers scraps together with table titbits (not ideal). However, at that time, there were hardly any vets in comparison to today, so dogs (along with cats and other animals) also weren't subject to constant or unnecessary flea, worm, or vaccination treatments, yet the average age for dogs was recorded at between 17-20, 17-20 years old 150 years ago, yet today it's around 10-12 at best!! What's gone so horribly wrong that we have reduced the life spans of these animals by almost half! Furthermore, we as a society have failed to realise this atrocity in the making!! As you continue to read, I will hopefully help shed some light on how, together with why this has happened and it isn't all down to bad breeding, we must realise that it's a collective however, some things play a larger role than others.

Sure4pets was established in 2014 and what a journey it has been so far, to date I have been researching for approximately ten years. The information I have been led to has been enlightening, 'eye opening' as the phrase goes and the above mentioned people (along with others that will have slipped my mind at this time) and who I have dedicated this book to have all been key to the information that will be provided, I will say now that much of the information I present, some of you may find hard to accept as I try to bring you out of this box, this indoctrination system, it may challenge some of your beliefs in approach alongside what is regarded as healthy foods in general and the approach to health. However, this is again down to the programming that society has been subject to. Hopefully, I can broaden your awareness, helping to open your mind, thinking with your own mind outside the box that we are placed in, allowing this new information that is actually old and in some cases ancient to be absorbed, acknowledged as well as understood, that to me as is the same with many others makes total sense, furthermore when it's applied brings theory to facts making it real.

The information that I will present for your perusal will hopefully bring enlightenment as well as inner standing, which will consist of the dog as a species, their SARF diet along with some of their characteristics. I hope it will help you better understand them along with why certain circumstances arise, we will also look at the body at a basic level. Furthermore, I will also cover the basics of biology - which in fact, should also show how this applies to all species, the basics of chemistry, how it applies to disease as well as again all species, what disease is, how it manifests, why it manifests, how to treat it – with real-life journeys proving the healing method but fundamentally how to help prevent disease in the first place. Finally, I will cover the true meaning of organic and inorganic, which again applies to all species whilst covering other subjects. These topics, altogether, are essential to truly understand how health is achieved in addition to why disease exists, but ultimately, they will pave the way to revealing the root cause! I will also identify the below three key areas that I have found are imperative and must be grouped together for us to truly inner stand nutrition, health, and disease.

1, The fact the body is electrical.

2, The basics of biology & Biochemistry

3, The basics of chemistry

Throughout this, I will repeatedly use what's known as the law of association, regularly referencing back to nature and using it to provide examples that should not only help you understand this information but retain it easier as you already have something to refer to.

Nature, as I say, is the best science lab we have; however, people are so far removed from nature that we fail to see the simplest facts of life that, when observed and broken down, allow easier understanding as well as application to help create along with mimic nature in a domesticated life.

When looking at nature, I'm taking you past the farmers' fields and the countryside beyond these manmade environments all the way back to the natural environment, where we find wild animals. This is where we find the truth, this is where we find the laws of nature, laws that don't have or require the constant use of synthetic or chemical treatments, cooked foods, biscuits, set meals with set times or set amounts, conditioning of soil to grow hybrid crops and this is where we find a creation that doesn't rely on the constant need for a vet or health care system designed to react to the problems created. Just the same as the birds that fly around our domesticated environment are also not subject to these constant unnatural or unnecessary treatments together with synthetic lab made "foods."

The dog as a species and it's SARF diet.

With so much conflicting information through various media channels, forums, raw feeding veterinary 'experts' at the forefront of the 'raw feeding' industry as well as 'raw food' manufactures. It is no wonder that many people are confused about what to feed their dogs, whether dogs are carnivores or omnivores or how to feed their dogs a raw food diet correctly, in order for them to thrive and live long and healthy lives just as "NATURE" intended for all animals.

There seems to be this huge assumption at the moment that dogs are omnivores which, as a matter of fact, still remains to be proven. However, we do have a plethora of very well-supported scientific, together with in-the-field evidence along with our own observations applied with common sense that proves dogs as a carnivore.

Dogs have been around for thousands of years, and although we have many breeds today, with lots of new breeds now present, they are all, in fact, the same species and are scientifically proven to be a direct descendant of the grey wolf. In fact, the scientific name for dogs is "Canis Lupus Familiarise," their ancestor the grey wolf, is known as "Canis Lupus" because by all scientific standards, together with evolutionary history (breeding approach), the dog is a wolf. A dog's Mitochondrial DNA is 99.8% identical to their ancestor, the wolf. MtDNA, in simple terms, is how the body processes its food allowing absorption into the cell, thus allowing growth, strength, regeneration, health, and vitality of the physical structure in its entirety at a cellular level.

Even in biological studies, wolves alongside dogs have been and are used side by side, so we have to acknowledge that although we have domesticated dogs as well as we have altered their appearance, giving them different breed names to visualise this, internally we have the mechanism of the wolf that functions the same meaning that we still see the same characteristics of the grey wolf along with natural innate traits seen but not realised in our dogs daily lives.

We can also use the animals' features, thus allowing us to categorise them; when we do this, we find either herbivores, carnivores, omnivores, or frugivores. If we start at the head, observing these features as well as anatomy, we find the following clear and distinctive differences between a carnivore, omnivore, or herbivore.

Dogs, as well as cats, still maintain their carnivorous features. They still have sharp and pointy teeth with claws designed to bring down their prey as well as to tear into the meat. Their eye position is still forward facing on their skull to focus on prey animals, whereas their prey have eyes set to the sides of their skulls to watch for attacks.

Focusing on the jaw structure of a carnivore, we find it's in a fixed position; it moves vertically up and down (like a pair of scissors). The omnivore, while on the contrary, together with the herbivore, have jaws that grind from side to side, dogs' jaws are in a fixed position, and they move vertically up and down. Next, we look at teeth; the teeth in our dog's mouth (like other carnivorous animals) are sharp and jagged, and their fourth upper and first lower molars (Teeth towards the back of their mouth where the most power in their jaw is) are in fact what we call carnassial teeth. The herbivore and omnivore have flat molars designed to assist with the grinding motion to help break down the vegetables and or grains.

Staying in the mouth, we then look at the salivary glands, the dog 'Canis Lupus Familiarise' produces just one single enzyme called lysozyme. Lysozyme literally lyses onto bacteria in order to destroy it because dogs aren't just carnivores; they are scavenging carnivores. They can consume decaying and sometimes rotting carcasses without having any issues with bacteria, this also helps explain and allows us to understand the old wife's tale 'if you have an injury or a wound, let your dog lick it,' the lysozyme helps to keep the wound clean from infection. It also explains why when the dog is out enjoying a walk loving life sniffing, licking (God only knows what lol), as well as marking their territory, essentially building their pee kingdom, when they return and lick our faces or our hands. We don't realise what they have been up to or even consider it, because the bacteria on anything they have had their face in has essentially been dealt with, so it doesn't affect us.

Going back to the omnivore and herbivore, we find there are two enzymes being produced from their salivary glands, amylase together with cellulose. These two enzymes kick start the breakdown of vegetables or grains, meaning that for these species, digestion begins in the mouth!

Moving on from the head to the digestive system, we observe that dogs have a relatively short foregut followed by a short, smooth un-sacculated colon. This means that food is processed quickly, and their digestive time is also generally between 4-12 hours (the 12-hr time generally required to break down the dense bone that is consumed,). The short colon, similar diameter as the small intestine, also limits the ability to allow for any vegetation or grains to ferment before digestion can take place. Vegetables along with other plant matter needs time to sit in order to ferment, which requires longer sacculated colon, which is usually found in omnivores and herbivores. The presence of a larger and longer small intestines and occasionally a caecum can provide a digestive time of between 12-14 hours. Although dogs do possess a caecum, it has no function.

Herbivores and omnivores possess a much more developed caecum which is used for bacterial fermentation of plant matter. Dogs have shorter foregut and hindgut, consistent with carnivorous animals. This is the reason why unprocessed plant matter is clearly visible in a dog's faeces when consumed, as there was no time for it to be broken down and thus digested. Therefore, the body hasn't taken that organic -living organism, broken it down to the mineral content in order to use the minerals to support itself (its cells), which is the whole point of digestion and what eating is actually about.

There are a number of very well-educated people that are aware of this who ignore these facts. They dismiss this observation encouraging people to feed "foods" that are not Species appropriate (and for many reasons, they know who they are), they tell you that vegetables and grains have to be pre-processed (blended or boiled) in order to allow your dog to get the necessary nutrition out of them, but regardless of how they attempt to manipulate digestion, we have to accept the fact that we are not feeding a SARF diet. If we were, our dogs would pose their own natural ability to process what is being fed and consumed on a regular basis and would, of course, be known as a SARF diet - (Species Appropriate Raw Food), not a raw food diet!

The dog's digestive system is simply not designed to break down plant matter which would allow them to extract any form of nutrition from them at all. Hence, we see it eliminated in their body's faeces and waste processing system in the exact form it was consumed, but it will tax the pancreas (I have experienced people through the shop whose dogs were diagnosed with pancreatitis whilst feeding copious amounts of vegetables), Other experts have also mentioned that these non-Species Appropriate Raw Foods interfere with calcium absorption. Another fact that I will cover later in the book is the starch base at the centre of most of the vegetables being pushed and recommended through the raw feeding community and in general.

The following is from the book "Wolves, Behaviour, Ecology, and Conservation" written by one of the top wolf biologists in the world! - L .D. Mech

Since a dog's internal physiology does not differ from a wolf, dogs have the same physiological and nutritional needs as those carnivorous predators, which, remember, "need to ingest all the major parts of their herbivorous prey, except the plants in the digestive system" to "grow and maintain their own bodies" (Mech, L.D. 2003. Wolves: Behaviour, Ecology, and Conservation.)

Over the past eight years, I have heard numerous reasons that lead people into the idea that their dogs are omnivores, these are however two misconceptions that tend to be used the most and that I have heard repeatedly. People, with these misconceptions, without realising are simply 'parroting' what they have been told, which is producing misinformation, it's the parroting of this misinformation without the ability to question that leads them to think their dogs need vegetation to achieve what's pushed as a "complete" diet in the form of what's also become known as a BARF diet– (Biologically Appropriate Raw Food). The word "complete" again is totally misunderstood as well as being a very misused word. The misinformation we are going to explain is also the reason people also feed what's now known as the BARF diet.

The first of these two misconceptions about the dogs being omnivores arises from the observations that "Dogs eat grass; grass is a form of vegetation, so they must be omnivores." Many people with this belief, are again, simply repeating information without questioning it from people with knowledge that isn't in its entirety, or people that have looked, but not observed to truly see. Let me take you back to nature, where we find all animals learn from observation followed by application. I always say a bird cannot learn how to fly without first observing followed by applying (we know there is a built-in ability), but all animals in nature learn by this simple law. This following part isn't intended to offend or take anything away from the countless hours people spend in what's become a precedent as education, and I'm not saying that all education is the same, but I see so many issues within this system as I view it with an open mind with the ability to question from what I see as natures perspective.

I see people sitting behind desks as opposed to observing and applying, I see an indoctrination system where people are given one-sided information coming from just one source. However, as pointed out, birds don't sit behind desks going over the theory of flying, with the seven-year course (for example) on how to fly, the degree or certification (a piece of paper) that follows, giving them permission to then take flight, regardless of a bird never actually observing or attempting to elaborate on this by actually putting it into practice?

As mentioned earlier in the book, I come from an engineering background; part of being a CI engineer also involved engineering gauges, workstations, etc., using equipment and machinery that required a hands-on approach whereby the constant use of such tools becomes second nature, as the body adapts, and muscle memory takes over. It means that things become automated, like driving a car, brushing your teeth, or driving the same route to work; this is the benefit of actual experience as opposed to theorising.

To give you an understanding of what I mean and what is happening, I can recall shortly before leaving my

Engineering position to set up sure4pets. The company I worked for had an influx of younger freshly "qualified" engineers with degrees to apparently prove competency, they had invested their time to learn passing their exams and were now deemed qualified by a system. These younger engineers with their degrees warranted the going salary due to their apparent and proven competency and why not, they are deemed competent. However, the problem was they couldn't do the job required as they didn't have the experience of physical work as they had only theorised. Take me for an example, I have been trained in-house by time served engineers, with over 150 years of experience between them, they taught me through observation and application (shadowing, or however you relate to this). These younger engineers, through no fault of their own, simply couldn't perform the basic tasks because almost all of their time had been spent theorising. Although they had spent several years in training, they had never actually done the work or experienced engineering in real life enough for it to become muscle memory, for it to be part of them, for it to be innate.

So with the potential that this book allows us to reconnect you with the awareness of observation and application or better put 'in the field experience or shadowing.' By using the example of observation with the ability to question, we address the first misconception actually observing a dog eating grass as opposed to simply parroting what we have been told or heard. We observe that dogs are selective with the type of grass they consume, choosing large thick blades; they tend to try and eat the first -4" and then move on, upon inspecting the grass, we find the first 3-4" is very abrasive. It has tiny fibres that are rough, almost like fine sandpaper; after the dog consumes this grass, it scrapes the intestinal walls. We then see the dog either induce vomiting, making themselves sick, if they don't induce vomit, we see them pass the grass in their faeces (as they allow it to pass through the colon) and in the form it was consumed. It makes it apparent that they are not digesting this as a food source, so are, of course, consuming it for other reasons. It's in the understanding of the body and how it works that we realise why! Which is, quite simply, to help clean their internal environment.

It seems necessary and important to point out that we as humans take care of our personal material belongings, house or car for example keeping them maintained and in working order. We clean the car inside as well as out, we service the engine, we clean the external of the body, we even clean the clothes we wear yet fail to consider the internal environment of the body, which needs to be cleaned and looked after more so than the external and our material belongings. Many animals have this natural inner standing and connection with themselves (their cells), but because people are so far removed from nature moreover with ourselves, we miss what's being presented due to a lack of awareness through critical observations. People then tend to make assumptions rather than observations; thus, in the instance of an animal consuming what could be a food source that is, in fact, a food source for other animals. We fail to understand that it could be and is, in fact using what has been consumed medicinally or to cleanse its internal system. Dogs, for example, are hard wired to consume grass, depending on diet and other factors they will do this often and naturally to help purge the digestive tract or their colon. I have also seen dogs increase the amount of grass they consume when fasting them, indicating that the fast has triggered their natural ability to assist the body in cleansing. I will make more sense of cleansing when we look at disease, and its cause. But I will leave you with the understanding that when we clean the car, for example, we use a soft abrasive sponge; this allows us to cleanse and pull the dirt out of the paint without damaging it; this is how grass works with dogs.

The second misconception also comes from the misinformation (believe me there is plenty of it within the raw feeding sector as well as in the world for that matter), and generally from people that are aware of the fact their dog is a wolf (on the basic level with regards nutrition and internal anatomy). Many of them will state that dogs must be omnivores because they eat the stomach contents of an animal; some people are told and even think that they consume the stomach contents first. Mainly due to a distortion of the information alongside the lack of ability to question themselves.

Although there is some truth to wolves and their descendants, dogs, consuming the stomach contents, the problem here is in assumption, assumption rather than a question. This is how the situation is being viewed by the observer, thus misunderstood generally through assumption because they don't have enough information to build on. They might have the awareness that dogs are scientifically proven to be descendant from the grey wolf, but they lack of having the bigger picture, including the knowledge of how the body works along with the cause of disease and the chemical processes, meaning that their overall evaluation is flawed from the start. This flawed misunderstanding is in the sense of Chinese whispers, we all know that as information has passed onto family or friends, details are forgotten or altered along the way, and is parroted. It's the inability to question (outside of the box) and think with our own minds rather than what's been programmed that leads people to think the situation is understood. Observation, as well as the lack of ability to question as opposed to just looking and or accepting (not humanities fault, it's part of what I have come to see as a program). So, coming back to wolves and or dogs eating the stomach contents, with a large animal, their stomach is actually large enough for the contents to be removed, yet with a small animal such as a rabbit or pheasant (for example), the stomach is too small so it's impossible to empty the contents resulting in the whole animal being consumed. This is the only reason the stomach together with its contents are eaten; it's generally said that the amount of undigested vegetation with a small animal and when consumed is between 1-2% which wouldn't cause any issues so it is simply passed as waste in its whole form, just like whole teeth have been seen in the faeces from a dog that's consumed a whole rabbit for example!!

This is what L.D. Mech has to say - in His book "Wolves, Behaviour, Ecology, and Conservation"

"Wolves usually tear into the body cavity of large prey and consume the larger internal organs, such as lungs, heart, and liver. The larger intestines [one of the main stomach chambers] is usually punctured during removal and the contents shaken out or spilled. The vegetation in the intestinal tract is of no interest to the wolves, but the stomach lining and intestinal walls are consumed, and their contents further strewn about the kill site.

This is from a guy considered to be one of the top wolf biologists in the world. So, with this information to hand as well as in mind, and particularly if you believe your dog to be an omnivore, you really need to be considering if your beliefs are built on solid foundations. what it should arouse are questions!! You should be making sure if your source was reliable, why was this information not in the mainstream or even on social media? What else are you not aware of?

As shown above, with one of the top wolf biologists in the world, it proves that most people are getting raw feeding (amongst many other things that I also aim to bring to light) wrong and for many reasons. Some we have covered, other reasons will be highlighted shortly, the key point to address now is not how this deceit has happened or to blame anyone; it's about seeing the root cause so we can rectify the problem. It is an opportunity to improve our dogs, cats, and other pets' lives by understanding what they should and shouldn't be eating by using nature, observation, the ability to question, application, and common sense, which goes a very long way. We must realise that we have been and are continuing to be disconnected from nature; hence many are getting things so very wrong.

With this in mind, I want to emphasise observing nature as our best teacher. Nature serves as the best scientific lab for making sense of many situations, including the understanding of a SARF diet separating it from the 'RAW DIET.' As it allows us to expose the key difference, again using nature to help us begin to look at what the true but moreover correct diet for dogs (a direct descendant of the grey wolf) is. So, within nature we find around a million species, billions of animals that live on earth; what we find with these billions of animals in nature is that they all consume a raw diet. The phrase "raw diet" is a well-known term within the movement of feeding dogs and has been for at least the past ten years and in particular the past five years, I have seen a significant increase in awareness. However, this phrase is a very open statement, I think that due to the awareness of these diets growing exponentially due to the visual improvement of health seen it has helped to provide more awareness to the benefits. Nevertheless, people have missed some fundamental basics when it comes to the real understanding of terms or words used when describing something, meaning that because of this boom in raw feeding, people are now taking to feeding raw foods to dogs that aren't part of their natural diet and for varying reasons as follows:

1: To make their dog's meal look special for their social media updates

2: Because they have seen others do the same (just because 10'000 people or more do the same thing) doesn't mean it's right? most people just tend to follow the crowd! Many in fear of appearing different.

3: Because they have been taught that a particular food source holds a certain nutritional value?

4: For monetary gain (you know who you are!)

5: General miss-information

So, in bringing your awareness back to the term "Raw feeding" specifically because people use it but don't acknowledge the fact that it's a very open statement. Many people, without realising, including nutritionists, are missing the very basics because of information that's coming through channels we rely on and has become an indoctrination tool.

Again, we have billions of animals that all consume a raw diet, this is one of the many laws of nature, but their raw food is what I call, and I have referred to already as a SARF diet. It is a "Species Appropriate Raw Food" diet and is specific to the species which has a unique digestive system for breaking a living organism down, allowing its body to utilise the nutrients to sustain itself (its cells). This is essentially what we referred to earlier as Mtdna.

One of the biggest issues I have observed and been presented with upon researching is that our current system is so lost in itself (by design) that it has forgotten and, in most cases, blindly ignores the very basics of how the body, a living organism works. It seems to have lost its awareness that in nature, we find Herbivores, Carnivores, Omnivores, and Frugivores; all these animals consume a raw diet with the key element that's it's a SARF diet. We cannot feed the SARF diet of a Polar bear to a Gorilla or vice versa, nor can we change their geographical location; that's how specific nature is and how seriously we have to take the basics of life and the true meaning of a SARF diet. **We are at a point where we are basically saying that we know the polar bear is a carnivore, but this grain or vegetable contains calcium and iron, or it contains "vitamin b12" and "protein," and as its raw, we can blend this and feed it to the polar bear! Or, in many cases, we can simply feed it anyway because others do! Can you see the madness?** This is how essential not only the right environment is to the health of a species but also the food source. This disconnection with nature and the body has significant effects on health, along with how our education system can and is leading us into a blind ideology of what's healthy and what's not. To observe the real connection to the SARF diet and its importance, we will be looking at the body at a basic level, how it works, along with the basics of biology to try to recap just what real nutrition is, how it works in reality along within nature on a basic, simple level, but first I want to continue to address the dog as a wolf.

Chapter 3: Understanding the dog as a wolf.

Having now covered the dog as a species with the focus being on their nutritional needs as a carnivore, we can now have a brief look at some important aspects of their characteristics that seem very important to grok, having had many people come to me with the same assumptions leading people into traps as I see. For example, with dogs refusing to eat, or with dogs who end up becoming what the owner generally sees as a "fussy eater."

One of the first things I explain to people during the discussion about their dogs' switching to SARF and if the dog/s will like or take to it- is "they normally take to SARF like a duck to water." In fact, what normally happens initially is that we see a very greedy dog, a dog that wants to eat as much as it can and will make a lot of noise to point this out, often begging for more, by jumping up at its owner, or moving their feeding bowl around.

When this happens, we tend to see people falling into the trap of assumption feeding the dog more food thinking the dog is still hungry, however after a few weeks, when the dog slows down and doesn't want to eat as much, they fall into the same trap of assumption thinking that the dog has or is going off the food. When in reality, the dog has actually slowed down due to the fact it has now realised there is a constant supply of this raw food.

As you will have grokked from reading this book, I often use the law of association to assist people understand things for what they truly are. Hence, I frequently refer to nature, so embarking on this journey and observing the fact that when there has been no food available for a lengthy period for a Lion, or a wolf, or any other animal for that matter, as soon as food does become available the animals tend to gorge themselves as if they have never eaten before. This is essentially what happens when most dogs are initially switched to their SARF diet due to the fact that for the first time they have been presented with real food, meaning that it makes perfect sense for them to overindulge (in reality and when fed synthetic foods prior to their SARF diet, they have never really eaten!). However with dogs as well as in particular with the domesticated environment together with the food on tap at regular times, after a certain time frame most people tend to find that their dog begins to take a step back thus isn't as eager or greedy as before, at this point and from experience most people think their dog is going off their SARF, initially their dog didn't know if their owner was going to feed SARF the day or week after? But once they comprehend it's their new daily feed, many will then only eat what they need to. The result is an assumption that they have or are going off the food.

What can also happen after a dog has been eating their SARF diet for a while is the development of what is considered a 'fussy eater!' What happens here is that their

44

dog becomes picky. This generally develops due to one of two reasons, first we have already covered, the second is more to do with the calculator used to work out a dog's rough daily feeding portion, which, has been around over 50 + years and is a very good tool to get dogs started with their SARF diet. It is only a guideline however and we often find that the daily portion suggested is too much so after a while the dog becomes selective, picking and choosing what meat types it wants to eat. Many owners assume that the dog is going off certain meats from their SARF diet as they begin to refuse to eat opting to select only specific meats, even though they might have started their SARF diet eating the whole variety initially. This, itself, presents the fact that they will eat the meat, at this point and in general you must realise that you're in control and not the dog. You also have to realise, and you will once you have read the fasting section further into the book, that a healthy dog will never starve itself. You must also accept that if you put a SARF meal down that, let's say, is duck and your dog refuses to eat, you don't have to frantically look for something else to feed your dog. Whenever a dog is refusing a meat type, the general advice is to place it down for 10-15 minutes of which after and if your dog has still refused to eat you take it back up, cover and then place it back into the fridge. This is repeated until your dog ascertains that there is no other food available; you also have to recognise that your refusal to back down and find something your dog will eat is not neglect. Its simply going back to nature whereby if the duck is the only food available and they hesitate, they might have to wait for another 3 to 5 days before food is available again and they eat, sometimes it's longer. L. D. Mech found with his in-field observations that wolves can go six weeks without food. Now, this is a worst-case scenario, but it shows us their capability and gives us a measuring point.

I always remember as a child, my mother would shout me for dinner or tea, and on many occasions, I either didn't like or want what was being served, or I simply wasn't hungry. Her reply to me as a typical Yorkshire Woman would be, 'thy either eats it kid, or tha goes wiout, cos thas now't else' I was out climbing trees running around frantic playing football, having lots of fun with bags of energy, my point is it never affected my health or my energy levels, these reasons will also be brough to light later in the book.

I also have personal experience with this and our Boy Oli who around 10 years ago was eating 1020g per day as per recommended with the original raw feeding calculator. After a period, he began turning his nose up at Chicken, Turkey as well as Duck, particularly, all the lighter meats. However, Beef, Lamb, Pork along with all the other bloody meats he would devour without hesitation. I observed that although he had days where he either didn't eat or ate less. His body condition never faulted, nor did his energy levels; in fact, he had more energy as did when I was younger. This showed me that although he was eating less per week than recommended. He was still getting enough food as his body condition was of an ideal shape. He had a waggy bum (Bulldogs don't have tails, lol) along with the 3 p's – peeing, playing as well as pooping. Furthermore, he was healthy and happy, which is why we decided to reduce his portion, decreasing 680g.Shortly after that, we found that he began eating the lighter meats again, why? because he had to, same as he would have to if He was in nature where the luxury of choice isn't available! This allowed us to provide a larger selection of meat types and keep His SARF diet varied.

Now don't get me wrong, when it comes to a SARF diet, although the most convenient method is to feed minced food, there are better and much more natural methods; however, the minces are still much more superior to the alternative. The main concern with minces and the 80-10-10 ranges mixes in particular is that these mixes typically contain the same sort of animal parts including muscle meat, bones, 5% liver, 5% kidney and maybe some heart which is still meat along with every now and then lung. However, many manufacturers get confused about what qualifies as offal. You see in butchery tripe as well as the heart is considered as offal; however, in truth, offal is anything that secretes, IE pancreas, spleen along with the brain, kidney, liver, and even testes, so if we look at this with awareness now understanding that the body is made up of trillions of cells, the cells in groups and the groups made up from specific minerals. We begin to observe that the complete diet, which will be covered in greater detail, is, ensuring we provide the 102 minerals that the physical body is made up of, with the added comprehension that the body doesn't age overnight. Hence the complete and balanced SARF diet is naturally provided over time, and not every meal like people have been programmed to believe. With this in mind as well as when we consider that the body is made up of around 102 minerals, it would be logical to feed whole prey. But it is important to comprehend that if that route was taken, the dog wouldn't necessarily need to eat every day because as you will discover further in the book, the primary energy source is oxygen, then water, and finally food. Thus, allowing us to provide organic minerals to support the regeneration of the body at a cellular level as and when the body requires, which, might I add, is dependent on what is consumed – IE thoughts, emotions, chemicals, synthetics etc. This is the reason why some people and animals look older or younger than others and essentially age differently!!

Traps that people fall into

Many people are being trapped and are being led into feeding foods that are simply not a SARF - Species Appropriate Raw Food, Kefir is one of many "Natural" products that are pushed as healthy, but we need be looking at this with the awareness of what food is and how nature truly works. For example, milk is a natural source of nourishment produced by a female to support the growth and development in the early stages of life and after birth. Milk not only provides essential minerals and nutrients for physical development, but the mother also passes on milk to support the immune system. Milk is also produced by different species for that species - IE cow's milk is for cows, dogs' milk is for dogs, human milk is for humans, and so on. So again, going back to nature (the best scientific lab we have), we find that no animal in nature consumes the milk from another animal, nor do they continue to consume milk as an adult (only Humans have been conditioned or as a better word, programmed to do this - which doesn't make it right, or healthy). Nature truly is the best scientific lab we have. We need to go back and look with an open eye and truly observe how it works thus to allow us to grasp on a level no truer than nature just what we should and shouldn't be doing with dogs (or any other animal) to create health and vitality with the real inner standing of 'we are what we consume'.

Now that we have established the dog as a species, their general nutritional needs, what we should look to feed as well as how we identify the dog as a carnivore. I now want to look at the species from a biological point. This is where we come back to basics, thus allowing us to truly understand what nutrition is at a biological level and more.

Understanding the body at a basic level and its function.

The understanding of the body at the basic level takes us right back to the very beginning, where it all starts from a single cell. This one cell multiplies into trillions of cells, at a physical level fundamentally it is ultimately what forms the physical structure of life, we then find two major vessels (blood) as well as (Lymph) these vessels which are elasticated pipe based systems flow throughout the body reaching every cell, there are microscopic cells, blood together with lymph vessels, these vessels are required thus are essential in order to (A) feed the body at a cellular level (which is actually all we are, or should ever be doing) in addition to (B) removing the waste not just from digestion but at a cellular level too (the waste should be natural-IE from a SARF diet). These vessels are both fluid based; the body is said to be around 70-80% water. Hence for the body to function with ease, the blood and lymph vessels must flow freely throughout the system.

Understanding the body's basic function as I have found is one of the key pieces of information required in truly inner-standing nutrition and health that I have come to realise on this journey. Furthermore, to achieve the goal with the ultimate aim, which is to prevent disease (dis-ease being the fact the body cannot function as easily as it could and in fact should) by understanding the cause (where the cure is found) in order, to achieve health, vitality, thus creating life longevity, in life.

The body, like anything that goes through a process, has a waste management along with an evacuation system; this in the body of a living organism is known as the lymphatic system (lymph). This system is just as, if not more important than, the venous system. Furthermore, it makes up a large part of the immune system; this is where we find the (B) cells and (T) cells. This system will be covered in more detail later in the book when we look at dis-ease as well as its many causes that fundamentally will actually come down to one simple factor that I have already mentioned several times.

However, for now, our focus is on the body. At its basic function, the human body consists of trillions of cells that make up its physical structure with only 2 major fluid systems, blood (venous system) and lymphatic (waste system and immune system). These systems, as mentioned, are fluid based, they have to flow freely together with efficiency in order for the body to function effectively but fundamentally healthily - just like a mechanical system, I.E an engine that has fuel flow to generate the system as well as oxygen intake allowing life to the engine as well as the exhaust to eliminate its waste, again we will cover this in the next section as we begin to learn about the disease, but essentially keep in mind that when the waste from any processing system cannot be eliminated efficiently, this is when problems begin to manifest.

When we look at the body, we need to be looking the same way that a mechanic examines and understands an engine. As an engine has a number of parts that all come together to form a structure that relies on every part present to maintain function, but in order for the system to function effectively and efficiently as it was intended, each part has to be in perfect working order so to maintain that working order we have to ensure that we use the correct fuel, the waste from the engine - exhaust can escape efficiently, we service the engine (clean the inside), ensure the correct grade of engine oil is used and that we don't over work it, these are all key factors to ensuring the system runs and operates as intended and for as long as possible.

Knowing that the body is simply trillions of cells with 2 major fluids, blood, and lymph, which are fluid-based systems, we can begin to appreciate that these fluid systems have to flow freely in order to maintain healthy function. There is an air intake that filters through the lungs before entering the blood, which is Iron (Iron essentially acts like a magnet in the body) pulling the oxygen molecule and the minerals extracted from a SARF diet to it. Thus, assisting in conveying them to the cells to help keep the body strong and healthy as it ages/regenerates). So, blood feeds the cells, and the lymphatic system (bodies sewer system and major part of the immune system) is how the body eliminates its waste (exhaust). The lymphatic system is said to be around 2-3 times the size of the venous system, it also has hundreds of lymph nodes (gates) that act like cess pits helping to break waste down which is then generally eliminated via the colon.

Looking at the body as a mechanical system associating it with an engine, in simple terms, we have pipes that supply fuel (to allow the engine to function) and pipes to eliminate the waste (exhaust).

The human body is equipped with several pipes that supply life and energy, allowing itself to support the regeneration of every cell that makes up the physical body along with pipes to remove its waste. One of the key parts of understanding this system is the awareness that many of these cells and pipes (blood together with lymph vessels) are microscopic and cannot be seen with naked eye. Therefore, they must be observed under a microscope. This is critical because it underscores the importance of not only a SARF diet but also ensuring that what we allow to enter the body has to be recognised, naturally to the system, and can be processed, assimilated, and eliminated, efficiently and effectively thus allowing health, vitality and ultimately life longevity to follow.

Chapter 4: The Basics of Biology and the True Meaning of Organic and Inorganic

Taken from the book "Herbology For Home Study" Written by Dr Edward Shook.

"Around 1874, a group of German, English, French and Italian scientists conducted an intensive study of the chemistry of the human body, principally by analysing the chemicals left over from ashes after incineration of particular organs, tissues and body parts, among these scientific investigators were: Dr Wm H. Schuessler of Olden burg, Germany; Dr Larbacher of Leipzig; Drs Grauvogl, Virchow, Moleschott, Italian; Dr M.D Walker, Scoth; Dr. J. T. O'Conner, English. The great French Scientist Alfred Binet (18th century) also contributed to our present-day knowledge of the Biological Chemistry.

Among the findings of these devoted and untiring physicians are the following:

(1) The osseous structure of the Human body is largely built and vitalized by calcium phosphate (57 percent), calcium carbonate (10%) and magnesium phosphate (1.3%).

(2) Brain and Nerves, by potassium and magnesium phosphate.

(3) Connective tissue cells, by silica.

(4) Elastic tissue, by calcium fluoride

(5) The blood, by Iron phosphate etc, etc.

These scientists and their important discoveries regarding the chemical composition of the ashes of these varying tissues laid the foundations and created the introduction of what we now know today as Bio-Chemistry – (The Chemistry of Life).

But Life is full of paradoxes and contradictions; and while we give these gentleman credit and admiration for giving us an important key to help solve the problem of disease, we know today that while they were correct about the chemical composition of the dead ashes, they were certainly in error to suppose that these inorganic cell salts, as they are called could possibly restore diseased human cells to life and health, through the administration of compounded inorganic lifeless matter".

This is the same with all and every organic life form (organic = a living organism = electrical= of life-A-live) on the biological level.

What had been discovered here was that the cell groups are composed of different minerals. In fact, the cellular structure is made up of around 102 minerals, making minerals the basis and foundations of life. Unfortunately, most people are totally unaware of this fact, and many people we rely on for health care don't realise because of the teaching system. Hence, we call them trace minerals. From my own personal development and discoveries, it appears that as time goes by, the teachings seem to be getting deliberately deprived of basic key information. Thus, creating deterioration throughout the approach to health care in general. We only need to observe what's been fed (as food) in all health care systems to see this.

We have essentially just established and confirmed what food is, by coming back to the basics of Biochemistry and it's understanding, having already covered what, in fact, I think most people are aware of but don't realise the real importance of - that the basis of life starts from just a single cell. This cell multiplies into trillions of cells thus it forms a full structure, this structure is what we call a living organism, whether human, dog, cat, fish, kangaroo etc, the physical construct in simplicity is just trillions of cells that are grouped together. These groups that form together are however different, meaning that we have a group of cells that make up the heart, a group of cells that make up the liver, a group of cells that make up the spleen, a group of cells that make up the bones, a group of cells that make up the kidneys, a group of cells that make up the pancreas, and so on and so forth. The main and only reason these cell groups are different in structure is due to the mineral make up. Again, we seem to have and be forgetting or rather not being taught when acknowledging the true basic principles of life, which are as follows; We live in a mineral kingdom, where minerals make up both living organism and the ground we stand on – ("dust to dust, ashes to ashes"). These minerals, however, are vastly different as shown and referenced above by Dr Shook. On one side, we have minerals that are in the form of a living organism with a positive charge and one's that are lifelessly found in the earth with a negative charge (ground), these are defined by 2 words "Organic & Inorganic." Before we look at these very important factors that help us truly connect the dots, we come back to the physical structure, that we have of course established at a basic level, is trillions of cells grouped together, and these cells are in different groups as pointed out because of the mineral make up.

The ageing process in the body of a living organism is influenced by various factors, including cellular degeneration and regeneration, which is affected by the rate and level of cell reproduction, the speed and extent of the ageing process is determined on many levels and includes, on a basic level, what is consumed, IE food, environment, thoughts, and emotions. However, what we are looking at in this book is what is consumed in the physical form (Matter) and not energetic (wave) essentially everything is energy, everything is frequency, vibration, and magnetism.

Every cell that makes up the physical structure relies on blood flow, nutrition, and lymph flow (IE, the waste being eliminated efficiently from the body). The cellular structure, when regenerating, relies on what is fed into the system, which is then processed through digestion and then at a cellular level to support self. For instance, in order to ensure we maintain strong, healthy bones, calcium, magnesium, and phosphorus are not only required but are essential. These are the food for the bones! the brain cells require carbon along with copper, the pancreas requires Chromium, and the blood is Iron (ion). Iron in the blood acts like a magnet pulling oxygen and minerals towards it, conveying them to the cells of the body. No amount of vitamins, omega 3's or 6's, or proteins are going to strengthen the body at a cellular level, purely and simply because the foundations of the cellular structure as a physical form (matter) are built on minerals. This is the basics of biochemistry and comes back to the fact that we live in a mineral kingdom that is, in fact, electrical. Yes the world that we live in (LIVE) is electrical; it has a-live (life) and an earth.

Organic and Inorganic

In this next chapter, I will be discussing the meaning of organic and inorganic. Some of you may wonder why it is necessary to delve into this topic. However, to allow one to observe the bigger picture at a simple level, we need all the information or, as I see, the Jigsaw pieces. We must realise that before something complex can be simplified (like a mobile phone, form of technology or biological system) we truly have to understand the makeup of it.

Organic:

Most words today, as already pointed out with the term "Raw feeding," are spoken and passed around without any real awareness or understanding of their true meaning, and I can't stress enough at this point how important it is to know their true meaning.

We see the same happening with what most people perceive as organic; many people are now of the belief that this means vegetables such as carrots, parsnips, strawberries. Many other fruits are grown in clean soil and or an environment that is clean and free of herbicides or pesticides, or that an animal has been reared in a natural and humane environment. In actual reality, the true meaning of organic is that it relates to life, living organisms and electrical. The body of a living organism is electrical so is the world that we live and exist in as previously mentioned, and we know that with electricity, we find a positive charge alongside a negative charge, "live and earth"; anything organic is alive – live and anything inorganic is dead – earth or ground as we know with an electrical circuit board.

So we have electrical devices such as ECGs that measure the heart rate and monitor the body's electrical frequency along with pacemakers and other devices such as defibrillators. The body is electrical; it is energetic. Thus, energy is measured in frequency; hence the frequency is transmitted through the device and is displayed. The world, as I mentioned, is electrical; hence, we see lightening in a thunderstorm; the ether is very much real (how can it not be?). It is also how information is sent from phones, radio, and television - through the energy ley lines/IE magnetic field; everything is magnetism, vibration, and frequency. Magnetism is a push-pull, a positive and negative complete circuit. It is a self-perpetuating energy field.

The body is an electrical system and is interconnected with mother earth. This is important to consider when understanding nutrition and what should be consumed, what is utilised, and therefore known as food through cellular assimilation. We do not simply feed the stomach or, as most people do, the hunger signal (including myself at one point in life).

Inorganic:

Inorganic means the total opposite. It represents something that is dead, lifeless, ground, and, in fact, earth. We cannot put something into the body of a living organism that's dead, void of a positive charge, void of energy and life and expect to get life from it, only certain life forms (on earth and in the ocean) - namely, trees, plants, flowers, grass and herbs, for example that grow from earth are able to take inorganic minerals (minerals with a negative charge) from earth to build their cellular structure. This essentially converts the negative charge to a positive charge and ultimately turns them into a liquid digestible organic and electrical food source so that when the herbivore (for example) comes along to consume it's SARF diet (plants), their digestive system, as per the species naturally breaks down and processes the organic minerals from that life form. In turn, using the organic minerals to support self as the body reproduces itself – (its cells) and regenerates using the minerals to strengthen the body at a cellular level, therefore providing strength in the physical structure; this is cell food;

this is real nutrition, this is real awareness and this is also how the carnivore (Dog) uses the cellular structure of the herbivore in order to support and sustain strength, health vitality and life longevity for its self. This is also the same as the herbivore does with its SARF diet and all other species, whether Omnivore or Frugivore. Remember, we live in a mineral kingdom with 2 forms of minerals = organic together with inorganic - live and earth. Hence the phrase "dust to dust, ashes to ashes"

Conclusion:

So with all this key information thus far and in mind we can begin to understand the dog as a species, what it's food is in the form of a SARF diet, what a SARF diet is, why it's key to ensure that we are feeding a SARF diet that's true to the species, and how it actually assimilates with the body to maintain strength health and vitality at a cellular level throughout the aging process. We also need to acknowledge and remember that what is consumed can also speed up the aging process causing the body to regenerate much quicker than it would do, meaning it's not food and is, in fact, acid-forming. We need to be conscious, thus considering foods that are consumed or fed to the animals in our care; we need to take on board this new information (that is in fact ancient and has always been true as long as carnivores, herbivores, omnivores, and frugivores have existed) and begin to understand so we can realise what real food is for the species in mind. Asking the question, "just because it's raw and holds nutritional value, can it actually be processed by the animal in question?" I.E are we feeding a SARF diet? I ask this question because I personally know that within the growth of the raw feeding sector, we now have around 80% of people that feed their dogs as omnivores and consider it a healthy diet. They are feeding all sorts of raw foods, and many are not aware of the real reasons they are feeding what they are or that it must, in fact, be a SARF diet. With dogs as a prime species in mind and what this book is essentially about, we not only have the science, as mentioned previously in the book, that shows us these animals fit into the carnivorous category, but we also have our own observations. Furthermore, we have already covered one of those observations regarding dogs and eating grass; we see the grass being eliminated in faeces in the form it was consumed because dogs do not process vegetation, and we see the exact same with vegetables (including Cruciferous) fed in chunks or whole forms, they are eliminated in faeces (via the waste system) in the form they were consumed (just like the blades of grass) as waste because the body cannot break them down in order to gain any of the organic minerals (life force energy) in order to support self.

Chapter 5: Challenging Our Beliefs

Staying in line with the SARF diet, we will return to nature. As mentioned earlier in the book I intend to challenge some of your beliefs regarding healthy foods, so here we go. It's the conscious observation with a truly open mind that allows us to see; this provides an awakened awareness of our environment, helping to provide a truthful understanding of what nutrition is, why a SARF diet is the only diet, and again, how we achieve true health and vitality through cellular assimilation to gain life longevity. let's take you on a journey, past the farmers' fields and the countryside looking at the following vegetable's that people are feeding their dogs because they believe they are an omnivore. As it's being recommended by others. I also want you to question where the following types of vegetables (including cruciferous) grow freely and or in abundance in nature –

Cauliflower

Broccoli

Cabbage

Sprouts

Carrots

Potatoes

Parsnips Green Beans

Sweet Potato

Garlic (not wild)

After seeing the list and asking the question myself, your answer will have been like my own, none of the above vegetables are found in nature. They don't grow freely or abundantly like vegetation and other natural foods do for the millions of species in nature that are herbivores or omnivores that consume plant matter. Upon observation, we may discover that certain foods grow well in soil that has been conditioned to specifically allow these types of "natural" foods (natural being another prime example of a word that is miss used and miss understood). to grow and flourish, these foods are what are known as hybrid foods, they were made in a lab (not nature's), different plant molecules are fused with a chemical called starch when starch is processed through digestion. It is turned into carbonic acid, which is one of the many acids that eats away at the mucus membrane that wraps around and protects the cell; alongside carbonic acid, is lactic and uric acid. The key point to take away here is that unnatural acid-forming foods damage the body at a cellular level; the continuing consumption of such hybrid and or acid-forming foods will, over time, lead to many health issues.

So if we want to come back to truly understanding the world that we live in (so we can identify real and true nutrition and what a SARF diet actually is) with the awareness that the world is electrical whilst considering the 3 major elements that makeup life otherwise known as the C, H, O arrangement – Carbon, Hydrogen, and Oxygen, we find that every food that is truly natural and comes from nature is complete in this CHO arrangement so what is achieved after the body has broken down its food source (a living organism = of life, electrical = live) is full assimilation into the cell. This is how a strong, healthy, and electrical cellular structure is achieved; this cannot be accomplished with hybrid foods, inorganic minerals, synthetic "foods," or chemicals and is a critical piece of information required when truly understanding real nutrition, health and how it's achieved on the biological level.

So now, that we have hopefully covered these basic understandings of the body, the world where we live and fuels creation through assimilation along with the food that forms real nutrition = organic minerals, we can have a deeper understanding of why a SARF diet is the only diet that should be provided to dogs. All species show us that nothing else has or ever will come close, we can now also address why everything else will and does over time lead to disease and in particular look at the effects that synthetic "foods" along with chemicals, additives, preservative as well as inorganic minerals added to these so called "complete and balanced foods" affect the body, by doing so we are essentially getting to the root cause of disease ultimately showing cause and effect, what we do creates either a positive or a negative outcome, so continuing on this road of understanding and coming back to helping cement the importance of a SARF diet and covering "what is consumed becomes us"- essentially health or disease, I want to again take you back to nature whereas already mentioned we find millions of species, billions of animals, with no cooking, boiling or blending found and certainly no biscuit (dried) or pre-cooked tinned foods, even Zoo keepers feed a SARF diet, you won't find a bag of biscuits that's states "complete and balanced!" in nature or in a Zoo. In nature, and as also mentioned, there are no chemical treatments – flea, worm, or vaccinations and nor do we see any of the above-mentioned used with birds that fly around our streets and neighborhoods. But yet they not only survive, they thrive without the need for so-called healthy necessary treatments. !? The only time nature has and does struggle is when we essentially start playing God and try to alter creation thus upset the balance (homeostasis) which is seen in many ways aside of what has already been mentioned as hunting, the use of technology that uses man-made electromagnetism altering the frequencies along with the natural vibration of nature known as the Schumann resonance, resulting in disease through the imbalance of vibration! whether the animal wanted it or even knew it was happening to them, but I digress this is another topic and not what My focus is about, never the less it links into what creates disease through awareness that everything is frequency, vibration and magnetism, essentially its why we need to be living together in the laws of nature or as close as we possibly can.

Summary

In one of the previous sections, "Understanding the body at a basic level and its function," we covered some important along with basic principles about the human body and its functions. First being that the physical body is composed of trillions of cells with two major vessels – blood and lymph. One vessel supplies the body with life while the other removes the body's waste. We covered the fact that there are microscopic cells, microscopic blood vessels, and microscopic lymph vessels. We are aware that the body is a fluid-based system, and to achieve health, flow is essential. We have also acquired knowledge that the body is electrical, being organic, and is, in fact, made up of around 102 minerals proven in the science that is biochemistry founded in the 1700s. We have also concluded that dogs are carnivores, and from all of this, we are able to deduce what we should be feeding and why; what we are now going to look at is disease together with how it is created which is generally described as inflammation, inflammation is believed to be the root of all disease and illness, it isn't, inflammation is symptomatic. Thus, the root cause is never addressed.

Chapter 6: Chemistry & Disease

First of all, chemistry applies to everything, and no matter what we look at, we will find either acidity or alkalinity; we can use the following to see how it's applied. For example, food is broken down by the body creating stomach acid (there is a natural chemical reaction created in the body from eating as mentioned previously!), the natural stomach acid breaks down what should be a SARF diet starting with the digestive process, just like when we cook food applying heat, we should be acknowledging that everything is chemistry, but cooking in line with nature is an unnatural acid approach because remember no animal in nature cooks its food.

We can also look at cleaning products, nail polish remover, herbicides together with pesticides, chemical flea and worming treatments and again find that these too work under the law of chemistry, either acid or alkaline; I'll leave you to work out which side of the Ph scale most of these work under but know today that we are living on the acid side of life! furthermore disease, as we're told, is caused from inflammation however the inflammation itself is a consequence of what has entered the body!. We need this understanding because we cannot provide the environment that the body needs to live in, which is homeostasis (a balanced pH environment, or simply put a chemical balance!) and expect the body to be able to function with ease as well as regenerate itself efficiently and effectively when using a synthetic acid or an acid forming approach, I would then ask you to consider the general approach offered to treat disease - with chemistry now in mind asking one's self if the approach used and recommended is in fact acid or alkali, or if it's organic = electrical, thus allowing it to assimilate with the body at a cellular level to either assist the body in cleansing at a cellular level/removing the cause, or assimilating to strengthen the cell structure, to promote regeneration thus leading to health or healing by providing the body with what it needs in order to heal itself – its cells alongside maintaining homeostasis.

I'm pretty sure that most of you are aware that acid is corrosive and although there are different levels of acidity we have to acknowledge what it does, a really good example of how different acidity levels affect certain life forms but still indicate what they do is looking at a common house hold product - washing up liquid, we don't see any immediate effects to skin after use and assume this is safe to use. However, if you take just a couple of drops of washing up liquid and add it to a 5 litre spray bottle and squirt a spider with this heavily watered down solution, the spider will die **(please, please don't do that as I'm not promoting it, just raising awareness about pH, chemistry along with its effects, take my word for it on this one).** I know this because it happened to me on a few occasions when I worked installing safety and security film to glass, which required a clean surface before installation, so although we barely see any effects from that acidity level with us or other life forms, it clearly impacts nature and the cellular structure of a living organism and is, in fact, devasting to other life forms.

When we talk about inflammation we are talking about an acidic environment and are entering into chemistry and the pH scale (Potential Of Hydrogen) which starts from 0 and reaches 14, a balanced body pH should be around pH:7 in order to maintain homeostasis/balance, above or below will cause disruption to the body of a living organism as the body struggles to maintain its chemistry (homeostasis) and when the body is knocked out of homeostasis, we will see disease manifest. It also creates an environment for certain and specific parasites to live in the body too (another cause of disease), being more specific it was noted by Dr Ian Billinghurst that with dogs fed a raw meat diet, stomach acidity was found to be between pH 1-2, stronger than hydrochloric acid, this pH level (acid environment) not only provides efficiency in the digestion of bone as it gets a repeated bath in this acid, but it also provides a barrier against parasites/worms and pathogens. However dogs that are fed cooked foods tend to have a more alkaline stomach acidity of between pH: 4-5 as the body adjusts it's chemistry, meaning that digestion of bone is much more difficult but also an environment in which parasites can build communities and essentially throw parties is created! Hence almost all dogs (and cats) that are fed cooked foods have to be wormed regularly, yet the vet (who is placed all their faith in their education and is oblivious in this area) tells us that feeding raw meat causes worms! I have to say, at this point, Our boy (Oli) is 12 years old. He has been fed a SARF diet for around eleven years. He is thriving with no skin issues; what's more, Oli has very clean ears along with beautiful soft fur. In addition to this, we have been told by many people He looks around five years old. He has had around seven worm counts in 11 years and never once had any issues with worms because His internal environment is in homeostasis! I deal with people in the shop all the time, and whenever we switch their dog/s to a SARF diet cutting out all unnecessary treatments as well as advising the owners to use worm counts (no chemicals), we tend to find that just like Oli, there is no evidence of worms! if they are new to SARF and a count reveals an issue with worms I will recommend the use of natural plant-based herbs to flush the worms from the body.

When we look at inflammation now, understanding its simply chemistry, We find that there are two categories when entering the acid side of life (which is where we are today, as mentioned) Chronic inflammation and Acute inflammation; chronic inflammation is, in reality, manmade and acute inflammation is a natural phenomenon the body uses to process a SARF diet as well as to heal itself and regenerate, both, however, are damaging even though one is necessary, you see although the body uses acute inflammation to process as well as to heal, we have to

71

comprehend that we are still wearing the system down as its using an acidic approach and essentially energy to repair itself – its cells, understandably there is a huge difference between acute and chronic inflammation. Moreover, there is also a big difference between natural acidity created in the body, synthetic acids entering the body as well as an acidic environment created from constipation and essentially a build-up of waste!

Chronic inflammation is where we find all major diseases – cancer, arthritis, diabetes, heart disease, liver disease, kidney disease, and skin disease etc.. Chronic inflammation is simply a result of what has entered the body "We are what you consume" – as I have pointed out, what is consumed does one of 2 things, it either assimilates with the body at a cellular level which is how we create and achieve health, vitality and life longevity for our dogs and other species, or it does the total opposite creating sickness thus over time leads to disease within the cell (which is what we are seeing today at an alarming level!) remember – "cause and effect" but be fully aware of its meaning, what we do in life with our dogs or with the body of a living organism, in general, will have 1 of 2 outcomes, it will either create a positive outcome or a negative (organic = positive, of life, living organism, electrical, inorganic = negative, lifeless, dead, ground, earth, are you getting it yet?).

Acute inflammation is where we find the body's natural healing ability. For example, cuts and lacerations heal through acute inflammation, along with a broken bone (the difference with a broken bone is that it has to be held in a fixed position, preventing it from moving in order to allow it to heal and repair– IE it has to fast!, we will cover fasting and its importance in the body's healing and regeneration shortly in the book.

Under acute inflammation, we also find the word "allergy," which is again another word thrown around by many without any real understanding. In fact, there is no such thing as an allergy, this phrase was coined around 1906 and didn't actually take a hold in society until around 1940. This phrase is used to cover a list of symptoms which are very much real and are listed below, but again, in reality, these symptoms are simply a reaction the body displays as a warning and is part of its healing process, the problem with the phrase "allergy" however is it removes us from the root cause and has an industry treating symptomatic! because when we look at the fact we find that the body uses acute inflammation to heal and we remember that "allergies" come under acute inflammation, we can acknowledge that the body's reactions are simply a sign that it's in a healing state, all due to what we have allowed to enter it.

Under the misconception and miss direction of "allergies," we find a number of symptoms/reactions;

Itching

Scratching

Rashes

Hotspots

Fur loss

Flaky skin

Dermatitis

Dirty Ears

Regular Ear infections

These symptoms (or, fault codes if we start to look at the body with understanding that it's like a mechanical machine) are the bodies way of communicating to us, it's a reaction whereby the body is essentially telling us that what has been fed or has entered it over a period of time (or recently) has caused constipation or is acidic, this creates a negative reaction, but in actual fact this is an opportunity to learn, if we actually observed to understand what the body is telling us which in simple terms is that the body is attempting to deal with it and what we should be observing with a greater inner standing, is just how this amazing creation (the body or should I say the living organism is, being the most advanced piece of technology on earth) actually works so we can become aware of these negative but necessary results that are being created and observed! by doing so we can then begin to see the root cause and not simply address the symptoms by reacting to the effects with lack of true awareness!. We need to be conscious that healing, by determining the root cause, cannot be created by addressing the symptoms but is in fact found when we understand the cause – cause and effect.

It is a basic understanding and acknowledgement in engineering that to fix a problem, the root cause has to be found; once the root cause has been located, one has to determine if the root cause can be improved so to prevent the issue from returning and is no different with disease or in fact anything else, I will touch more on cause and effect shortly.

Skin & It's Connection To Understanding What Most People Know And Are Told Are Allergies As Well A Link To Disease

Skin is, in fact, an organ and, generally unknown by most, is the largest eliminative organ filter on the body; hence it is often referred to as the third kidney! It is supposed to eliminate as many toxins, mucus and gases per day as the lungs, kidneys and bowels do. Skin conditions, in general, are simply a sign of the elimination process taking place due to the effects of incorrect foods, additives, preservatives, drugs etc., that create constipation within the body, clogging up the body's waste management system (ultimately lymphatic) and resulting in the visual symptoms such as scratching, rashes, dry, flaky skin, hotspots, dermatitis, fur loss etc., these are then considered as 'allergies' through these conditions, we can then also find issues with parasites which are scavengers and are found anywhere toxicity and dead cells are present, they live on top of and in between the layers of the skin, all these symptoms are considered as a disease.

Having more of an understanding of skin, the fact it's a filter, as well as the symptoms observed from what is, in reality, constipation creating inflammation (chemistry), We can begin to Grok that most issues with dogs and other pets start off as 'allergies' meaning that the body is reacting - ultimately attempting to heal from what has been allowed to enter and all 'allergy' symptoms can be identified as an acidic state due to constipation, for example –

1. Scratching is the result of waste/toxins being eliminated via the skin; these waste/toxins are acidic, hence the scratching symptom! – to understand this on a deeper level, consider the reaction from a burn; shortly after, it becomes irritated, and the urge to scratch is produced.

2. Dry, flaky skin is simply dead cells; again, acid is corrosive, and the result is dead cells; the visual symptom is dry flaky skin.

3. Dermatitis is an acidic condition and, in fact, cellular degeneration and regeneration as the body ends up in a cycle due to an acidic state.

4. Fur loss or excessive shedding can be explained by inflammation or, moreover, an acidic state as the hair follicles are affected by the acid being eliminated via the skin.

5. Baldness or bald patches again is an acidic state, whereby there is more constipation in local and specific areas of the body resulting in dis-ease of

function, meaning that the body cannot function with ease due to constipation (build-up of waste that is acidic) thus the cells are damaged due to acid being corrosive, we also have the added contribution that every cell in the body first and foremost requires oxygen to function efficiently.

6. Regular dirty ears signify stagnation of waste in the head area. Moreover, in the lymphatic system and in particular shows that the lymph nodes are congested – constipated, thus the body, in its amazing wisdom, seeks to push the waste out through other orifices. In this instance, it's easier and more efficient for the body to eliminate this waste through the ears.

These are many explanations of what is actually happening when a so called 'allergy' is diagnosed however inflammation moreover constipation is linked to the same issue and generally because the root cause isn't being addressed or understood, nor is the cause being removed, due to lack of awareness most people including the poor vet don't understand what's happening or why thus the very approach required is missed and we then carry on with no regards to what caused the issue in the beginning as well as continuing to cause the issue, what proceeds is symptomatic treatment whilst having no idea of cause, the result is and can only be chronic disease and an early death, yet with the information provided along with the acknowledgement of "We are what We consume" we can begin to look at dealing with the symptoms which are simply the body's reactions, with the ability to look at the root cause of the problem by acknowledging what has been going into the body, as opposed to masking the symptoms which is simply preventing the body from healing and in fact fighting against the body's innate defense mechanism.

The skin isn't just a filter for eliminating; it's also a sponge and is used to absorb, meaning that toxins can also be passed through and into the internal environment causing the above symptoms that can be and often are diagnosed as an "allergic reaction." However, the symptoms or rather reactions most often take time to manifest as they are processed through the system.

The skin, being a sponge, also breaths as all cells do and thus needs oxygen. An example of this would be to look at someone who is bed bound. They have to be turned so to prevent bed sores (cellular degeneration through lack of oxygen), which is a perfect and visual example that oxygen deprivation to the cell is what creates disease and highlights very clearly that if the blockage isn't external and is, in fact, internal, we will and do see what's often diagnosed as skin disease! This understanding will become more apparent further into the book when we look at the two theories of disease, but I have seen first-hand when the body is toxic, resulting in skin issues as well as skin disease, all because the cells have broken down, or are breaking down through lack of oxygen, and in actual fact because of constipation within the body (lymphatic or venous system). This is the same with any other chronic disease! The cells can't eliminate the waste due to lymph stagnation; thus, the degeneration process begins. When we get to the approach I use with dogs it is unique and one that to date no one else is applying as a specific and direct approach, this approach however is nothing new or unique as it is used by many in treating people today and has been many times in the past, when applied we begin to find examples of how we deal with the disease at its root, thus allowing the body the opportunity to begin to heal itself – its cells.

This approach, however, is only found when looking back in time, searching away from what I see as the mainstream programming machine!

Cause & Effect & Disease

I have mentioned many times so far throughout the book that 'We are what we consume.' This gives us the causation of disease (which manifests over time); what I would like to point out more so, is why and how!

The "cause and effect" model is known as the Newtonian model. It looks at the fact that what we do creates 1 of 2 outcomes, either a positive effect or a negative effect, whereas "creating an effect" (in this instance, creating health consciously with awareness) is known as the quantum model, my aim is to bring people into the quantum model where we truly inner stand that we can create health with our dogs, other species and self through knowledge of the body

– Biology, Biochemistry, Chemistry and what organic and inorganic truly identify, you see there is no real difference when we look at life as a living organism and at a cellular level, meaning that everything covered in this book can actually be applied to all other life forms including Human, and in fact, is and has been. Knowing what you know so far, which model makes more sense to you?

Before, when I was a Continuous improvement engineer, I couldn't fix and then prevent a problem from returning within the production cell if I hadn't found the direct cause; once the direct cause had been determined, we then, if needed looked to build in quality control (so looked at understanding why the problem had occurred and how we could prevent it) to ensure the cell functioned efficiently without the issue returning! Consequently, disease within the body and essentially the cell (cellular structure) – the disease is no different.

We are now at the point of cause and effect, remembering that we are told "the root of all disease is inflammation" – however, in actual fact, inflammation is caused by constipation, and constipation is the effect and consequence of what has been consumed, IE what has been allowed to enter the body, I cannot stress the importance of the simple phrase 'WE ARE WHAT WE CONSUME' because this paramount phrase truly is the direct cause of either health or disease, however as mentioned its part of a bigger picture that must be combined in order to truly inner stand!.

By now, one might be thinking, well, how does Constipation link in with a dis-ease such as Cancer, which, from my understanding, is uncontrolled cell mitosis which has two forms 'congestion and degenerative'? Both accumulate from the same cause. However, one is simply congestion in lymph, and the other is a result of congestion backing up into the cell leading to mucosa being discharged to help fight the inflammation (an immune response). If the lymphatic system is stagnant, the mucus cannot be eliminated efficiently, which prevents the amount of oxygen from reaching the cell. This leads to weakness and, ultimately, cell death. This cycle then continues and develops further due to the same cause, constipation from what has been consumed and, in most cases, still is, what also happens in most cases is the treatment provided is one that is in the form of an acidic approach. I will ask you at this stage if it makes sense to you to treat a disease that is created from an acidic condition with an acidic approach. Or if an alkaline approach would be more sufficient and effective.

Hopefully, you will now understand that Inflammation is caused by constipation, but what I would like to delve into more is how. This is when we come back to the lymphatic system - the body's sewer system and a major part of the immune system, that if you remember is said to be at least 2-3 times the size of the venous system. This sewer system has hundreds of lymph nodes. Furthermore, it has microscopic sections therefore, when this sewer system cannot efficiently process or remove the waste from what has been consumed efficiently, constipation will be the result which can and does affect the cell and cell mitosis, which in fact is due to lymphatic stagnation, constipation can also be identified as blood clots and the cause exactly the same- 'we are what we consume.'

Inflammation is simply acidosis. It causes cellular degeneration because acid is corrosive. We can begin to acknowledge this phrase on a deeper level alongside the fact that "we are what we consume." These unnatural substances, synthetics, inorganics or chemicals that are either acidic in nature or acid-forming, mainly cause lymphatic stagnation, "constipation" (think about tumors or growths, which are simply blockages in the lymphatic system-elasticated pipework network) these are all a result of the fact the body is struggling to process something it was never designed to, however regardless of whether we actually see a growth or tumor all most all disease in simple terms is just constipation. We even see the same issue in the blood vessel with clots, as mentioned! It's stagnation IE – constipation it prevents flow which will lead to disease and ultimately a major problem as the oxygen (main life force) as well as minerals are prevented from reaching the cell.

Inflammation, however, as I have already pointed out, along with constipation, are, in fact, still symptoms, because when we actually get right back to the root cause (cause and effect), we come back to the phrase I am repeatedly typing "we are what we consume" because as already pointed out and mentioned what enters the body even when injected simply does one of 2 things:

1. It either assimilates with the cells because it's natural; thus, in turn, it strengthens the cell, which results in a healthy physical structure because its natural, the body knows how to process it in order to eliminate the waste efficiently as well as effectively so is removed as quickly as possible via the lymphatic system thus is finally evacuated via the colon, this efficient system is what creates a strong, healthy cell resulting in a strong physical healthy structure, or

2. It does the total opposite because the body struggles to process what's being fed, and the blood and or lymphatic system is affected. The blood, along with the lymphatic system, then becomes sluggish or stagnant, resulting in the processing together with the waste evacuation system slowing down in many instances for example, it backs up, causing clots in the venous system or it backs up into the cell from the lymph causing cellular degeneration through acidosis.

We can again use the law of association, looking at the house in that we live (just like Dr Robert Morse does) using the bathroom as an example of one of the trillions of cells within the body, with the toilet being the lymphatic vessel coming from the cell allowing elimination of its waste so to help us better understand allowing us to acknowledge the lymphatic system together with how it backs up creating disease over time.

The toilet is used to eliminate our waste; it is, however, designed specifically to eliminate faeces, urine and toilet paper, which is also designed to breakdown in this system in order for the system to be able to process besides managing it effectively with efficiency, however when people decide to attempt to flush something like a baby wipe – foreign to and through this system at some point it's going to get stuck, or the system is going to struggle with it because it doesn't breakdown as the toilet paper does, nor was the system designed to process this foreign object in the first place. The baby wipes generally then get lodged. This could be 20 to 50 yards into the sewer system, maybe more, maybe less, but once stuck, the normal waste that this system was designed to process cannot pass efficiently. Thus, it slowly begins to build up.

We see similarities between the sewer system and the body's lymphatic system; when we consider the lymphatic system is connected to every cell in the body and every cell is connected to every other cell in the body, the sewer system (world lymphatic system) is connected to every house on the street and every house on the street is connected to the houses on the estate and at some point the system comes together at a waste plant, like a lymphatic node/gate (in the body) which acts as a cesspit in essence and further breaks the waste down so it can be processed and dealt with efficiently – **all the best designs and ideas come from nature!**

So this wipe has been flushed down the sewer system but has become stuck, and nothing other than the normal waste (faeces, urine and toilet paper - as designed) has passed through the system. However, the normal waste cannot be processed fully as it's stuck behind the foreign object (the baby wipe), so it slowly begins to back up until you begin to see the "symptom" of the toilet becoming blocked, which might take 2-3 months at which point it begins to affect the bathroom (cell) and in general there is no correlation between the cause and then effect because of the time delay! you're then left wondering how this could have happened? The blockage took all that time to build up into the toilet that's in the bathroom (cell), and if we continue to use the toilet, ignoring the fact there is an issue, the issue will remain. If we then continue to use the toilet ignoring the symptom, it will overflow and spill out into the bathroom (the cell); this is essentially what happens in the body (on a basic level), we have to acknowledge that the blockage might have taken two months to manifest, but there was no awareness of what was happening because we couldn't see? Again this is what happens within the body and is why we hear the phrase "you are what you eat," The effects of what has been consumed can take months and sometimes years to manifest, then when the symptoms appear, we generally mask the symptoms with drugs continuing to consume (or feed) the same things that lead to the cause of the issue's in the first place thus because of this the actual cause in almost every case is missed so then without realising we don't see that the issues are created from what we have allowed inot the body, the result is dis-ease! This is why in just 150 years, we have, as mentioned, seen the average life spans of the dog as a species reduce from 17 to 20 years to around 8-10 years, with the disease becoming rife, resulting in the growth of a veterinary industry!?

Considering anything that doesn't derive from nature IE, anything that isn't specifically part of a SARF diet, should not enter the body of any living organism. If it does, it will, over time, have some negative results on the system as the body struggles in its attempt to process and eliminate it via its sewer system unless it's dealt with.

Keeping our focus on sewer systems whilst coming back to the body's own sewer system and essentially the waste it produces and has to process from what has been allowed to enter it, the principle is exactly the same, and as already covered, there are only two sides to chemistry with the body's waste being acidic!, so looking at the lymphatic system that is having to process foreign matter (synthetic = fake "foods") along with synthetic chemical based treatments as well as atmospheric chemicals from the likes of candles, plug-in air fresheners and more, is it no wonder we see so much dis-ease as the bodies only vessels (blood and lymph), the major processing as well as waste eliminating system (sewer system and immune system) struggles to cope with this attack on its operating system and waste begins to back up in the lymphatic system and mainly through the filtering organs kidneys and liver (groups of cells with two major vessels).

The Theories of Disease

There are two theories to the cause of disease. In the 1800's Louis Pasteur, a French Chemist, theorised that germs (microorganisms) are the cause of most diseases, and this theory became the most popular in determining the causation, this, in turn, paved the way for antibiotics (antibiotics kill both good and bad bacteria) along with vaccines that seek to prevent single diseases. Physiologist Claude Bernard, however, who was a friend of Louis Pasteur, was teaching and explaining the terrain theory and, in fact, said that the terrain, along with its condition when becoming weakened by deficiencies or toxicity, will become ill when exposed to pathogens, this explains why some people become sick when exposed to the same pathogen, and some do not, it was this reason Louis Pasteur admitted that "Bernard was right: the pathogen is nothing, the terrain is everything."

The terrain theory can generally be explained by using the law of association and more specifically the environment of a fish tank. This is a contained environment and comparable to a cell of the body; the body in of its self is a vessel and with this awareness as well as the understanding, we can begin to make sense of dis-ease.

Within the tank, we have a fish swimming around that, of course, is fed, which results in waste being created; thus, the fish defecates in its environment; the faeces and urine produced by the fish is evacuated from the body but remain in the contained environment, this waste as mentioned is acidic, meaning that if this environment isn't maintained IE; if we don't keep it clean the chemistry (pH level) is altered! This will result in the fish becoming sick. The general approach and reaction to this today is to medicate the fish using a barrage of drugs including antibiotics as well as to vaccinate as per Louis Pasteur's approach This approach is symptomatic thus by treating the fish it isn't acknowledging the root cause and if we simply maintained the environment - ultimately the cleanliness, chemistry or rather homeostasis would be achieved, and health would be maintained!, this is achieved by looking at and understanding yet again the cause!.

So again, when we go back to nature with the awareness around 1 million species, billions of animals on earth all live by the laws of nature, consuming their SARF diet with no cooking, boiling, blending, biscuits or unnatural chemical flea, worms and vaccination treatments! And we remind ourselves that we also don't see the disease in nature like we do in domesticated animals or with people, We begin to discern its simply because the wild and natural living animals have clean tanks (vessels), and because they only consume their SARF diet they support their body at a cellular level, hence nature does not need a vet because there are no deficiencies or toxicity within their vessels like we see with dogs and cats. Birds that fly around our streets don't have the need for these constant treatments or care, and again around 150 years ago we barely saw a vet in sight, dogs were fed butchers scraps along with table titbits, on average their age was recorded at between 17-20 years old, now it's around 10 years old, now we see vets on almost every high street and we are pushed all these treatments along with biscuit "Foods", other cooked or processed foods, and not only this, people have to make regular visits to their vet because the main issue isn't understood, nor is it dealt with, it is rather masked then made worse as more unnatural synthetics alongside chemicals are fed into the body thus preventing the body from displaying it's problem (a fault code if you like, like we see on the modern engine), the result is we fail to see that what we have been allowing into the body has over time created a problem that is essentially displayed as a symptom, so again when we look at the phrase "We are what We consume" accepting its importance using the law of cause and effect with the terrain theory in mind which can actually be applied logically and is in actual fact evident as it links directly into inflammation, we can now begin to see the most direct cause to dis-ease today, we can also deduce that the body is giving us warning signs that we should seek to learn from by observing with a questioning mind in order to work with the body looking at the cause, additionally we should consider that this also includes what enters the body through the lungs as well as through the skin remembering skin is the largest organ filter, but is also a sponge, we can start to see on a very basic level the origin of dis-ease with the understanding of chemistry and how the body works at a cellular level!.

I always say to my customers as well as people that come into the shop wanting to switch their dogs to a raw (SARF diet), "We need to go back to nature" because we're so disconnected, we can't even see the obvious truth to Grok where we are going wrong! Nature and its laws should be heavily observed and applied with these understandings!

Conclusion

Hopefully, you are now beginning to see that the key to health for our fur babies (and life in general as a living organism, something that is electrical) is knowing that what we consume (or put through the body of the living organism) will only have 1 of 2 outcomes, either health and vitality or disease and illness, both are created over time and when we arrive at that state of either dis-ease or health!?, at this point we continue to see the same state manifesting due to what has been consumed and entered the body until we alter the approach!.

In almost all cases with the disease today and as mentioned, the cause (what is allowed to enter the body) is masked, and the symptoms that the body presents are hidden! This approach will only further lead to more disease as time passes and as we continue with the same approach which caused the symptoms or disease in the first place, rather than acknowledging that the body is actually telling us what we have been allowing to enter has had a negative impact and is causing a reaction/problem! alongside this we also have to understand the fact that the reaction and or disease that follows is generally delayed and takes time to manifest, meaning that causation can be and is again almost always missed.

This book is about providing as much awareness and understanding as possible, so as to help prevent disease with our dogs, interestingly and as I'm sure and hope you Grok by now, it's the same with all life forms and by ensuring we get the diet along with the environment right for the body, both internal and external! This, as mentioned, is where the cure is found.

Essentially if we are to truly inner stand disease at a basic level and what is being witnessed, in most cases, it's down to just two main factors, as already mentioned – weakness and toxicity; weakness is the result of oxygen deprivation and lack of minerals being fed to the cellular structure, as also stated earlier in the book and when acknowledging biochemistry, the trillions of cells that make up the physical body are in groups, and the groups of cells are separated by the mineral content. Again, wrong food selections, synthetics, hybrid foods and such will not lay the foundations for a strong, healthy cell or allow the function of the body's system and will, over time, lead to weakness as the body not only struggles but as it ages and regenerates itself becomes weak, the wrong selections of foods. Or allowance of unnatural and foreign substances (flea, worm vaccinations, etc) will also lead to the second factor 'toxicity' which also affects cell health, lymph, as well as blood flow, leading to constipation, which can even be parasitic, parasitic however generally links back to the chemistry of the body, whereby the environment is created for them to thrive, it's even said, and I believe that many parasitic issues are miss-sold as a virus and the parasites actually hide behind heavy metals that have been allowed to enter the body through vaccines and other atmospheric sources!.

Evidently, dis-ease is simply a lack of oxygen to the cell. We witness first-hand the effects of when observing anyone that is bed bound and with no one turning them, what precedes are bed sores (referred to as pressure sores, but is, in fact, cell breakdown due to oxygen deprivation); left long enough these sores will contain little worms that manifested from the degeneration/death of the cells in that particular area, every cell in the body first and foremost requires oxygen to maintain life and function of ease.

Just before we move on and begin looking at and understanding how we approach a dis-eased state that will allow us to assist the body in healing, let's remind ourselves again that the body heals itself because many people have forgotten and blindly look through what the body actually does as well as what it's capable of, not through any fault of our own, but because we simply are not told or given this awareness.

I see that most people are kept so busy today with jobs, bills, raising families and what we're all guilty of sometimes – "keeping up with the Joneses" along with generally having this rushed pace of life racing through the days to get everything done, that most don't have time to think, particularly about the simple things, which are normally the most important, so we go through life aging, just like our dogs and other domesticated animals do and end up lacking these simple but so necessary facts and understandings to life that I have mentioned that would help us to achieve the highest of riches in any life that we could want and hope for, FOR our dogs and in fact all life which is "HEALTH".

Chapter 7: Fasting And Its Association With Healing

Throughout the ages as well as still in nature today, fasting has been and is taking place. It has proven itself to be the most efficient way for the body to heal by allowing it to rest. We see the body initiate fasting when and if we become very sick and animals in nature also apply this basic yet supernatural spectacle initiated by the body required for recovery allowing the body to heal itself – its cells. Moreover, we have also identified previously that in nature there are no set meals, set times or set amounts, most animals in nature fast all the time.

Because there is more information coming back to us about the powers of fasting, we are also seeing numerous scientific studies being conducted Again!! - that also shows the effects along with the proven benefits of this amazing as well as natural phenomenon.

Although there are many that have usedand recommended the use of fasting, there are four people that spring to mind for me when I explain fasting to others in order to create the understanding of what I call the foundations of healing- Mr Hippocrates "The Father Of Medicine" Professor Arnold Ehret, Dr Robert Morse and Alfredo Bowman – AKA Dr Sebi.

Mr Hippocrates, in and around 365-BC cured every disease known to man at that time. His methods included fasting and the use of herbs "The herbs are for the healing of the nations," as the phrase goes, we will also cover some herbs briefly later in the book, their powers, and benefits, but for now, we will continue with the foundations of healing – which as mentioned is fasting.

Mr Hippocrates is known for creating the system of medicine that is used and known today. People who work in this field are still under the Hippocratic oath, unfortunately however and in many of the approaches to medicine besides treatments today, none are following His teachings, nor do they understand the approach or the body because if they did, then they wouldn't follow or continue with the approach now taught in the schooling system!

Mr Hippocrates isn't just known throughout History for His healing abilities or as the Father of medicine. He is also known for many quotes; however, at this point, there is only one I want to detail –

"To eat when you are sick is to feed your sickness."

When we look back at what we have just covered with the terrain theory, Biology, Chemistry and essentially Biochemistry in mind, it's easy to see why fasting is important alongside how it's so effective. We can't expect to cleanse the system (cells, blood, and lymph) in order to remove the cause of disease if we continue to burden these systems by making them continue to work! If, alongside this, we also acknowledge that the body is a waste-producing machine producing waste at a cellular level – around one hundred million cells per day, again we can begin to Grok the importance of reducing the amount of processing the body has to do at a cellular level in order to allow it to operate more efficiently and with ease.

Professor Arnold Ehret was a German Naturopath who wrote a book called "Mucusless diet healing system" He published His book in 1938. Like many others that became and did become advocates for fasting cured himself of a disease known as "Brights Disease" – (inflammation of the kidneys). He did so by learning about as well as applying fasting and the approach, He had but tried almost every other approach, and they had failed Him. After allowing His body to heal itself, Professor Ehret began helping others, He actually opened up a sanatorium where people could access this natural approach to healing and recorded the effects alongside the findings He made, He mentions in His book that He recorded many more successful healing journeys whereby the body was free from the dis-ease in its entirety, although I wonder if these records are available or in fact still in takt!?.

Professor Ehret also recorded His own experiences of fasting, talking about how much more energy He had, even when exercising with friends who were consuming what was regarded at the time as a healthy diet finding that in many cases, He was actually outperforming them, even though He was fasting! I can also personally vouch for this extra supply of energy, having personally introduced and applied regular fasting in my life today and, in fact, completing a 3-week fruit juice fast. What I also find when fasting on raw foods and fruits is I have more mental clarity along with focus, it's incredible!

I was introduced to Professor Arnold Ehret around two years ago (2021) after watching and essentially revisiting one of the many videos Dr Sebi made that can be found on YouTube, I tend to revisit books, videos etc., as the more our awareness grows, the more you see, and We tend to see things that We had missed before when revisiting them, I had missed Sebi talking about this book and its author, and felt it was worth exploring.

Dr Robert Morse was raised in Indiana on a diet that consisted of refined sugars, grains, meat, and dairy products, the result for Him was constant issues with congestion and blocked sinus cavities, and at one point in time, he was addicted to nasal drops, this condition leads him to severe constipation, bleeding haemorrhoids alongside this he would suffer from migraine headaches every three days or so, to top this off He was also obese due to His diet! He was taken from one specialist to another with no success in the removal of the condition. However, in the 60's He became a raw food eater after discovering Ehret's work amongst other natural healers, healing himself of all conditions. Dr Robert Morse introduced me to the lymphatic system alongside its function, He has studied the lymphatic system for over 40 years now, and I believe He is the most experienced and knowledgeable Man on the subject. He has also healed many people of disease and promotes fasting, He himself fasts and in fact in His book 'THE DETOX MIRACLE

SOURCEBOOK' talks about His personal experience with fasting.

Alfredo Bowman – AKA DR Sebi was born in Honduras in 1933 with an Asthma, a condition seen throughout the world today. However, by the time He was 30 years old, He was overweight, diabetic and had become impotent. It was in his search for an answer to his impotence that he was introduced to a Mexican healer "Alferdo Cortez "who, after first of all finding out what Sebi's diet consisted of, then had Sebi Fast on fruit juice and herbs for 90 days, every dis-ease Sebi experienced before the fast was reversed through this process, from this He decided to dedicate His life to learning about the body, natural health and diet, becoming one of the todays best unknown healers of all time. Over a period of around 40 years, Dr Sebi referenced both Hippocrates, Arnold Ehret as well as many others when teaching people about healing and the tools required to assist the body along the journey. Sebi produced many videos explaining various issues with the approach to the treatment of illness and cause of disease. Thus, he Himself assisted many people on their healing journey, succoring many in removing their disease with the use of fasting, along with herbs and fruits. For myself, alongside many others, Dr Sebi simplified healing, bringing so many truths aside from common sense when observing the body, chemistry, and regeneration.

I think it's important to note and point out that Professor Ehret, Dr Robert Morse and Dr Sebi, alongside many others, re-discovered fasting alongside a more natural approach to health as they simply weren't getting the results of health and healing, they felt they should and needed from the mainstream approach!! It's also important for me to state that I can concur with their claims, having read of and personally seen many cases where the dis-ease had and has been removed through applying the approach of cleansing the body at a cellular level (cleaning the tank), with the use of fasting and herbs whilst also revitalising the cells with minerals. Essentially re-balancing the chemistry within the body – bringing homeostasis back to the system.

I personally have been describing fasting as the foundation of healing from my own awareness and inner standing for the past three years, so as you can imagine, when I read Professor Ehret's book and found that He describes fasting as the master key, I was amazed at the similarities, but how else do you describe fasting once you know how it works?.

To help bring more insight into why I describe fasting as "The foundations of healing," we can again use Nature alongside the law of association to show that fasting is also a proven method of healing and is, in fact, nothing new as it has always been there. However, it's not been in our awareness, but as the saying goes and we mentioned earlier– "there is nothing new under the Sun"!, meaning that we are simply re-discovering what already exists and has been used in the past.

Fasting and its necessity in assisting the body to heal can be grokked when perceiving a broken bone within the body. Let's say the elbow is broken, for example, and whether the break needs to be repositioned, pinned etc. or not, we can begin to see where fasting is used to initiate, thus allowing the body to heal itself because in order to allow it to heal, and heal efficiently and effectively, it is generally placed in a sling (or a pot) and rested (FAST) from any movement for between 6-8 weeks!.

This fasting period allows the cells to heal; any movement would either slow down the healing process or prevent it dramatically, thus compromising the effectiveness and efficiency of the healing operation!

This understanding of healing within the body is no different from any other issue that needs to be healed. How can the body heal if we continue to work it? Again, we arrive back to chemistry but with the added element and introduction of energy when exploring further how fasting works and the power of this marvelous tool.

I think most people realise that the body creates stomach acid, stomach acid breaks down a food source (there are only 2 sides to chemistry) and in order to help the body gain access to the minerals that make up that organic life form (Ideally and naturally being a SARF diet), acid is generated and a chemical reaction results in the body being able to breakdown what has been devoured, the cells then process, meaning the whole body is working, so inflammation through digestion has kicked in, the body breaks down a food source in order to support self at a cellular level, moreover it then has to process and eliminate the waste in the form of faeces, and urine, which are acidic, throughout all of this the body is using energy to achieve this whether it truly needs to or not, so how can the body truly heal itself when in using this mechanism a natural inflamed state has to be undertaken, What I will cover next is how energy and the digestive mechanism can be better used to cleanse the body of anything it doesn't need, showing that when the body goes through the digestive process whist in the need of rest, cleansing thus ultimately healing, it is in fact burdening the system causing further illness or dis-ease allowing Mr Hippocrates statement above to make more sense.

Association Of Energy, Fasting And Healing

If and when we can grok (understand something intuitively or with empathy) the fact that the body is electrical and essentially energetic, we also begin to understand that energy plays a major role in healing, considering that the body uses energy on so many levels, aging, whereby the body replaces 100's of millions of cells per day, breathing, physical activity, brain function and digestion (to name the most obvious) it's easy to grok why fasting again is imperative to healing, as we start to free up energy, giving the body less work to accomplish.

Once more, we can use the law of association to show how energy is used through digestion with animals, in general, that gorge or simply feast, eating too much in one sitting. What is observed afterwards is a resting state as the body physically becomes lethargic, and the animal generally falls into a sleep.

We even see this with Humanity when overindulging and essentially feasting, resulting in tiredness and what I have often heard referenced as a "food coma," leaving the body with an enormous amount of work to carry out and what does the body require to process the small mountain of food consumed, energy!, meaning that the energy that was available before the feast for physical activity is no longer accessible due to the fact that this energy is sucked inwards and the body is now in a lethargic state due to the amount of work it now has to undertake!

We often see the same lethargy in sickness and or disease and, in particular, a healing state due to the fact that the body's energy is being sucked inwards to try to regenerate and maintain itself; again, I have seen this numerous times with dogs. In the shop, when they are brought in, IN a diseased state! and in particular, as their body begins its cleansing alongside its detoxing process in order to bring about healing.

Detoxing

The sole purpose of a detox is to purge toxins such as chemicals besides heavy metals along with environmental elements from the body by helping to create the conditions allowing the body to turn them into waste. The goal is to enhance the body's detoxification pathways (primarily the liver) as it's the main detoxifying organ.

Detoxing involves a change in diet, but more importantly, lifestyle. There must be a total switch from one approach to another, essentially one that's more in line with the body and its requirements. Detoxing can also include the use of certain herbal teas used to assist the body in the detoxification process. Physical activity can also be key as this is how we pump the lymphatic system, which also plays a major role being the actual system moving the waste through the system and into the liver – cells with two major vessels!

Cleansing

The key objective of cleansing is to clean out the body's sewer system (lymph) from the digestive tract (which is the goal of the dog when it consumes grass, as already pointed out, grass however, won't cleanse through the cell) as it won't enter the lymphatic vessel working through the cells, including the liver, kidneys skin, blood etc., remember, the body is simply trillions of cells with two major vessels. The cleansing will allow the elimination of impacted faecal matter, parasites, and fungi, all the result of constipation within the sewer system from what has entered the body.

When cleansing and as part of the detoxing process too, we have to ensure that we eliminate all unnatural substances entering the body (through change of lifestyle and ultimately approach) we must ensure there are no chemicals, synthetics or even none SARF foods being ingested. This includes milk or any related dairy products. We have to again acknowledge what should as well as shouldn't be consumed, not just unnatural "foods" but also foods that are specific to the species. Besides this we should also understand what would be consumed at a certain age or up to a certain age, like mothers milk, and then never again! The simplest way to achieve a true SARF diet for our dogs is to ask oneself, "What would my dog eat as a wolf in nature" Then ask, "What would my dog find naturally in the wild." If what you are considering giving isn't within the realm of these two questions, then the question has answered itself, If you don't know that answer then seek to find it, you can find lots of very helpful information at www.sure4pets.uk.

Throughout the detoxing and cleansing protocol, fasting is, of course, key and, as pointed out earlier, as I see is, "The foundation of healing" and, as Professor Arnold Ehret stated, "The Master Key." With extended fasting periods as well as determined by the type of fast used and required, we can also see the body enter the stage of autophagy. The effects of this can be seen in the appearance of a fever whereby the body kicks up heat and in particular inflammation in order to destroy weak, damaged or dying cells along with anything else in the body that doesn't belong in the body, such as tumors, growths, parasites and toxins in general.

With the understanding that the body of a living organism is electrical (hence it's organic), we cannot expect efficiency in healing, nor can we really expect to see the body regenerate itself (its cells) effectively, especially if the body's energy is being spread out to cover physical activities, digestion and then also trying to heal and in particular if we're not removing the cause by continuing on the same path that created the problem in the first place.

There are many approaches to fasting, and depending on the approach taken, it will determine the body's natural as well as its relevant response, fundamentally a fast will allow the body to begin reducing inflammation through rest; at this stage, we can sometimes witness the elimination of stomach acid which can be observed and is generally known to many as "hunger pukes" (yellow bile being rejected), if this is seen it generally settles after 2-3 days, but can take longer as the body begins to reduce inflammation and essentially begins to deal with the battle between acidity and alkalinity - lost homeostasis (chemical imbalance) that creates dis-ease). Effectively and due to the fact, the body isn't having to work to process food, we are providing more energy for the body to focus on cleansing and the regeneration of its cells thus ultimately healing.

When given the opportunity to fast (rest), the body can begin to utilise as much of this freed energy gained as possible, enhancing the healing action and due to the fact it's an amazing and efficient system, it will try to do this as quickly as possible, consequently, the approach the body intuitively takes can differ depending on how many cells are damaged so need to be replaced as well as the location of the issue, one of the main benefits but moreover super tools the body can initiate when fasting is autophagy.

Fundamentally, healing and regeneration is often seen in the form of a symptom and can be scary to see, to say the least, in numerous occasions the symptoms become worse before improvement is witnessed as the body sets to work on its healing mission!, what's also important to note at this point is that we have to remember that it is known that trillions of cells make up the body (around 75 trillion for the human structure) every cell is connected to every cell through the venous and lymphatic vessels, as well as this when we recall the fact "we are what we consume" reminding ourselves again that what is consumed becomes us, meaning that the trillions of cells can only be as strong and as healthy as what has been consumed and once we begin feeding a SARF diet as well as going about cutting out the causes of disease (synthetics, chemicals etc.) besides implementing fasting, the body is going to start to detox as well as cleanse thus essentially we launch its healing ability and begin this necessary journey, but not only are we effectively flushing toxicity from the system, the body will also - if given the opportunity or if necessary begin to replace weak, damaged or dying cells which will further burden an already compromised lymphatic system and is essentially what also leads to intensified symptoms of dis-ease as the filtering organs such as the liver, kidneys and colon struggle to cope with the demand!.

Autophagy, as mentioned, is one of the body's many natural modalities that allows it to regain homeostasis in order to effectively go through a healing process to achieve health once again. All the symptoms of illness are one and the same and are the body's attempt to heal, simply presenting "cause and effect" which in fact highlights that drastic changes need to be made and symptoms understood.

Fevers are today as all the body's natural defence mechanisms are, acknowledged and understood to be a negative reaction and something that shouldn't be occurring, this in a sense is true if we grasp to acknowledge that all health issues are, in fact the direct result of incorrect foods, chemical toxicity and imbalances! However, natural reactions should be allowed, and trust should be placed back into what I see as the most advanced piece of technology on earth (the living organism – the body). This amazing biological structure is, in fact, prevented from its attempt to heal, and what ensues is a battle between the body's natural defense mechanism, the direct cause and symptom suppressing drugs.

As mentioned before, fasting also gives the body more energy to focus on healing, a perfect example of energy and its importance, which is something that came to my awareness recently through the amazing work of Dr Joe

Dispenza, is when we look at stress, fear or even anxiety and how these energy affect the body, again I mentioned this briefly earlier and wasn't going to include it, however, I feel it is necessary to help bring awareness of energy and its importance to the understanding of how it ties into healing and ultimately health. I also feel it's important to bring awareness to the fact that everything is energy with again only two sides – positive along with negative and how these energies impact but, more importantly, benefit the body's natural regenerative cycle or prevent its regeneration. This is also paramount to understanding health and dis-ease!

It is a scientific fact that stress, fear, as well as anxiety weaken the body, particularly when re-occurring. There is a combination of reactions to these emotions (which are negative emotions) which trigger what's known as the "fight-or-flight" response. The fight-or-flight response provides all animals with a burst of energy so that it can respond to perceived dangers (in the external world). This enormous amount of energy and overproduction of stress hormones (chemical messengers) over time plays havoc on the body, disrupting almost all the body's processes and causing major issues internally (particularly if the threat is coming from the mind) because, if you remember, the body is always a construction site, using energy to remove weak or damaged cells replacing them with new healthy cells (aging), the body in actual fact goes through millions of tasks per day (all requiring energy internally, without any conscious awareness from the brain), so when the body is stuck in this state, most of the energy the body requires to function as an organic living electrical organism is actually being lost externally!.

It is also a scientific fact that the emotions of happiness, joy, gratitude, and a feeling of wholeness or freedom (positive) trigger hormones like dopamine, serotonin and, for example, oxytocin. These all benefit the body by helping to boost its natural immune system.

With this awareness of energy in mind, we can begin to see just how important fasting is energetically by giving the body less work to do and, in most cases, a well-deserved rest. It also comes back to what I mentioned earlier and again goes back to nature, where we find that fasting is a natural phenomenon and, in fact, one of the laws of nature, animals can only eat when food becomes available. It was noted after being observed by L .D. Mech that Wolves can survive without food for around six weeks before they become weak, provided they have access to fresh, clean water, "6 weeks!" and most people begin to panic if their dog doesn't eat for a day or 2. Why? - because of the lack of awareness that has consumed society today alongside the social programming that we have to eat, eat, eat! leaving most people vulnerable to the fact that when it comes to the hierarchy of food and its importance to life and health, it has been placed at the top of the ladder.

My yearning is that you can now see how wrong this is with the awareness gained; in actual fact, health isn't and should not be measured on the amount of food our dogs or any other animal consumes, but rather on their body condition, a waggy tail and what I call the 3P's – peeing, playing and pooing, although less food generally means fewer stools, that said we could sometimes see an increase in faecal matter being produced when cleansing as the body removes the waste it hasn't been able to, this may be visualized as mucus, dark stools, loose stools and very smelly stools.

The Fight!

Before we come to a conclusion, fundamentally the end of the book, I would like to try to point out '**The Fight**' that we're up against not only in altering the mentality in showing people another side to what they accept as the only approach to dealing with the disease through lack of awareness but of course that causation is also part of that fight, by this I mean truly assisting people in the realisation that the only thing that should be entering the body is what nature intended and not what has become a president or is not directly from nature. I also want to point out something I Grokked myself recently – the actual fight the body is in due to what has been allowed to enter it by which, in fact, displays the very symptoms seen as illness or dis-ease! but then the fight that follows against the body's innate defense mechanism as it attempts to carry out its job.

Through the shop, I get to see many of our Fur customers; thankfully, most are healthy and are thriving. However, we do get people who have issues with their dogs (but are still using chemical flea, worm, and vaccination treatments), so unfortunately, due to today's approach to what is deemed healthy besides necessary in an industry that is thriving! We are still seeing health issues that we shouldn't. There are also the people that are badly miss-informed and switch their dogs to raw then, as the dog's body begins to cleanse, we see the toxins rise to the surface, beholding the cleansing process taking place, which as mentioned, is not recognised for what it is thus is seen as an illness and due to the fact that most have no idea of what we have covered in this book there is no understanding of what is actually occurring or why. Therefore, the result is, of course, a trip to the Vet, most Vets begin by asking what is being fed, and more often than not and as soon as the owner says 'raw,' most people will be convinced to put their dogs back onto biscuits in addition to treating the symptomatic issue thus suppressing the body's natural healing ability. I have witnessed first-hand with many dogs whose bodies have been so dirty internally that we see the toxicity spilling out through the skin as the body struggles to cope and, in particular, generally the kidneys & liver. The visual results are extremely distressing. Furthermore, the suffering that these poor animals endure is unnecessary; many simply started out as "allergies" or as we better know now "acute inflammation" - the body's natural healing ability, merely doing the innate job it was designed to do because of what has entered the body!!, this whole approach taken is what results in what I have termed "**The fight**" against the bodies innate ability to protect and heal itself – its cells is created!.

When it comes to providing the body with what it needs to heal itself, there are as I see a number of fundamental keys required to achieve these desired results

1. Understanding of the body, along with the cause of disease

2. Grokking the natural approach required that will allow the body to heal itself.

3. Faith (belief) in the body's ability to heal itself along with the approach.

4. Fasting

5. Ensuring the correct herbs are used so to assist the body on its healing journey (extremely important)

6. Patience

7. Persistence

These seven keys are essential in attaining results when it comes to healing; these keys if followed would also create the cure through prevention. However, and as mentioned getting people to think outside the box allowing them to see through the general paradigm is part of "**The Fight.**"

When I have a dog owner that's on board with my approach but moreover has faith in the approach without the frustration of how long it might take to deal with their dogs' disease or illness, together we are able to over time, cleanse the body at a cellular level through the age-old method of fasting, ensuring that we aren't putting anything into the body that we shouldn't, alongside this with the use of specific herbal tonics We assist the body on its cleansing and healing journey, the body is then able to heal itself, the body is its own healer, all we have to do is create the environment!. Initially, sadly up to date it is apparent to me that most people only tend to be fully committed when they have nothing to lose, IE, when they had been told there is nothing that can be done to save their dog, this as you can imagine, makes it much harder to reverse the damage through the natural approach, generally taking much longer due to fact that the body is forced to push the toxicity deep into itself (at a cellular level) that in of itself results in trillions of cells becoming weak, damaged or dying. Thus, the work required to attain health can be a long road, but not impossible to arrive at that destination of healing. Now however, I think due to the fact we are gathering more evidence from the healing journeys, having assisted a number of dogs to date with minor issues, I am gradually starting to see more people take the information on board and are also applying it with faith as they have seen real examples which as I see helps in My aim, which is to get people to grok the cause so we can prevent these issues through conscious awareness! Furthermore, if I can also help you begin to understand the body with how it works, we might be able to place more trust as well as faith back into this marvel of creation, thus actually putting an end to working against the body (**The Fight**) but rather work with it.

I would like to share with you part of a message conversation between the owner and a breeder. However, I only have the owner's reply, but it's an example that gave me a deeper inner standing of "**The Fight,**" this came from a customer who is a responsible breeder, always producing healthy litters and has been coming into the shop for around five years or so now. The lady sent me the following through; between the message below, I will be interposing to help try and identify what's happening, thus bringing to light 'THE FIGHT' –

'Hi all, I hope you are all okay. We are having a horrid time with Boston. He had some sickness last Thursday and was sick with blood on Friday. He was due his booster (as He occasionally goes into the kennels). Since then, he has had to have two days stay at the vets (Sat and Sun) and is now back in today for x-rays and ultrasounds as they can't get to the bottom of what is going on.'

He had loose poop on Thursday Morn and didn't eat all his breakfast. He was eating grass and being sick (grassy bile) two or three times on Thursday afternoon/evening, so we didn't feed Him Fri morn either he was sick again, but it was brown bile with flecks of blood. He did have a 24hr fast. On Fri his temp was 39.9'

Let me explain what's going on here! Sickness is simply the body's primary method for flushing something quickly from its system (it is not, I repeat not a disease or illness!!). This is the same when diarrhoea is witnessed, too. We also begin to see the body initiate an innate fast as Boston is given a short fast.

We have had, prior to these symptoms, a puppy that has received its initial inoculations! - remember cause and effect?

We then witness the puppy eating grass due to the fact it's attempting to cleanse the internal system (we discussed grass earlier in the book along with how as well as why a dog will consume it)

We also see the owner provide a short 24 hrs fast that will give the body a boost (by saving energy) to deal with the issue. We also witness the body begin to create a fever empowering the body to burn what it's struggling to remove! This is the body's natural defence mechanism at work; what follows will hopefully be identified as 'THE FIGHT' on this system without realisation; hence – 'they can't get to the bottom of what is going on'. as stated above by the vet to the owner!.

'He had an anti-sickness and anti-bac injection. By Sat he hadn't drunk or eaten anything and wasn't peeing, so

115

went back to the vets' (**His body has initiated a natural fast**)*'-temp still 39.9'* (**This is the body is FIGHTING!**)

'they kept him in on a fluid drip. Temp came down to 39.1, so they sent him home and asked to see him the following morning.'

The anti-sickness drug will prevent the body's innate response to flush, preventing it from naturally removing what it clearly needs to! Creating constipation! Antibiotics have also been given (based on the germ theory) that not only attack bad bacteria but also destroy good bacteria; a dog is born (like a Human) without an immune system, it continues to develop and grow as they do. It's said that a dog's immune system is fully developed at around seven months old, yet they are given a drug that will damage and is known to damage natural immunity. Hence Dr's are dubious today about giving antibiotics.

'After the anti-sickness and anti-biotic injection, He continued to be unwell and not wanting to eat (**Because His body is trying to defend/protect itself and is being hindered with more unnatural toxins**)*, so went back to the vets Saturday and Sunday. On Sunday, they gave Him more steroids, and He had a short period of feeling better but went downhill again Monday afternoon and yesterday, so back to the vet this morning. He seems to be very stiff and uncomfortable when they are looking at Him. His Lymph nodes were enlarged over the weekend but not so bad today, although they are still enlarged – but His temp was 41.3,*

116

they have taken full blood, and the only thing showing is raised white blood cells. I'm hoping it's a very bad virus, and He's starting to feel better by the weekend.'

What can be witnessed here is the battle! Boston has already had synthetic drugs given to Him to treat the symptomatic issue. However, all this does is prevent his body from doing the innate job it is designed to do, however, what's very clear here after knowing about the lymphatic system and chemistry (acid and alkalinity) is that lymph node swelling is due to the fact it's backed up, why is it backed up? – because it's having to process something that it was never designed to process, and the body is struggling, hence it kicked up another fever at 41.3 degree's so it could burn what it couldn't cope with, the stiffness and pain are also due to the back up in the lymph caused by what has been allowed to enter the body – cause and effect!' I would also point out at this stage that the raised white blood cells are also indicative of an immune response too! Boston's body is working incredibly hard at this point but is losing due to the plethora of drugs fighting to prevent the symptoms. The symptoms are the body's natural defense mechanism in action. What can be Grokked at this point is the initial issue is not only being suppressed, but they are adding to the toxicity, and the body is being forced to push it deeper into itself – its cells.

These next two sections are also part of the message the breeder shared with me. They were, as you can imagine, very

117

mixed up, so I have tried to make sense of the order, but again they show clearly the problem that we were up against!
_

'Since Then, he has had two days at the vet (Sat and Sun) and is now back in today for x-rays and ultrasounds as they can't get to the bottom of what is going on; they thought a bug then a virus. He's had blood which came back fine other than the raised white blood cells but nothing else. He had a short relief from steroids but is now again running a fever of 41-degree temp. He's not really eating! Just had a call from the vets as they are unsure what's going on but are worried that a young dog isn't improving with symptomatic treatment, so are now talking about meningitis, autoimmune or worse, cancer. Waiting to see if the x-rays or ultrasound show anything today.'

If you have understood what I have discussed so far about blood and lymph, you will also see the problem and total waste of time in testing the blood, because the issue as in all cases today is in the lymph. *As soon as he got there, they suggested that He may have **idiopathic poly arthritis and/or steroid-responsive meningitis arteritis**. He has all the symptoms when I've read up on it. He was really in pain and uncomfortable around his wrist joints and neck, and when they examined Him. He's had a CT scan and samples taken of His joint fluid.*

Boston def diagnosed with idiopathic polyarthritis. He seems to be responding well to the steroids, and the vet has said he's a lot brighter today.'

I am aware She is covering the same issues, but there are a few key issues that need to be brought to light and to people's awareness. Everything up to this point has been an attack on the body's natural immune system, with no understanding whatsoever of the cause or the body's innate and defensive response! The poor vets have no idea what's going on (that's not only clear in the above, but they have also told this to the owner), so the obvious problem here is that they are talking about a number of potential issues creating fear and are blindly throwing their artillery in the form of steroids, x-rays (radiation) CT scans (Radiation) antibiotics (stress hormones), Ultrasounds fundamentally responding as well as reacting to something they don't know what they're responding to and are in fact causing further symptoms as they knock the body out of homeostasis and vibration – remember the body is electrical, it is a frequency, everything electrical carries a frequency so what damage has all the radiation also caused, or will cause later!?

I want to point out a few words, their meanings along with associations that have been used in the above as I'm sure people don't really Grok the meaning of them, which creates a problem with sight and understanding of again cause! So taken from the above –

119

'He may have idiopathic poly arthritis and/or steroid-responsive meningitis arteritis.' The keyword that I want to focus on firstly is 'responsive.'

Responsive meaning-

reacting quickly and positively. I agree that the steroid has created a quick reaction, but I think it's safe to say that it's not a positive reaction!

What are the synonyms of responsive?

Responsive

- active.
- aware.
- compassionate.
- conscious.
- **reactive.** – 'showing a response to a stimulus.'
- receptive.
- **sensitive.** - 'easily hurt or damaged'
- **susceptible.** – 'likely or liable to be influenced or harmed by a particular thing.'

The next word I would like to look at is 'Idiopathic.'

Idiopathic meaning-

relating to or denoting any disease or condition which arises spontaneously or for which the cause is unknown.'

I think we have covered enough in the book up to this point to have some form of an educated along with a discerning understanding of the cause.

The last two words I would like to bring to your attention are 'meningitis' and 'arthritis'.

Alfredo Bowman, AKA - Dr Sebi (one of the best unknown healers of our time), said that all dis-ease is a result of the mucous membrane being compromised from the consumption of acid-forming substances- 'you are what you consume.' Professor Arnold Ehret also said the same.

Dr Sebi said that when the body becomes saturated with acid poisons, the body will suffer from one or more mucus disorders.

- *Mucus in the stomach = gastritis*
- *Mucus of the mouth = stomatitis*
- *Mucus of the throat = diptheritis*
- *Mucus of the nose = rhinitis*
- *Mucus of the bronci = bronchitis, hayfever, asthma*
- *Mucus of the lungs = pulmonitis*
- *Mucus of the eye = conjunctivitis*
- *Mucus of the ears = otitis*
- *Mucus of the brain = prenitis also meningitis*
- *Mucus of the small intestine = enteritis*
- *Mucus of the large intestine = colitis*
- *Mucus of the appendix = appendicitis*
- *Mucus of the liver = hepatitis*
- *Mucus of the pancreas = pancreatitis*
- *Mucus of the kidneys = nephritis*

- *Mucus of the vagina = vaginitis*

- *Mucus of the uterus = metritis*

- *Mucus of the ovaries = Ovaritis*

- *Mucus of the bladder = cystitis*

- *Mucus of the prostate = prostatisis*

- *Mucus of the Heart = myocorditis*

"He had a short relief from the steroids the vets gave him but is now running a 41-degree temp. He's not really eating ☹ just had a call from the vets as they are unsure what's going on but are worried that a young dog isn't improving with the symptomatic treatment, so are now talking about meningitis, autoimmune or worse still, potentially cancer."

They gave Boston steroids when what immunity He has at the point was already at work dealing with the issue, steroids are known to offer short relief, but the issue always comes back. The question needing to be asked is why, Hopefully, by now, you are starting to Grok this) His body (lymphatic system) then had the synthetic steroids to deal with and on top of the anti-sickness drug too. 'He's not really eating' No, His body has put itself in a natural fast because it's already struggling to cope with processing!!, The fever is also generated when the body needs to deal with something quickly as the body attempts to burn what doesn't belong there. It's at war! As mentioned above. 'They are unsure what's going on' - they are battling against the body's innate defence mechanism but have absolutely no idea because they have been taught with a symptomatic approach; they don't Grok the body, how it works or understand cause and affect!! They have also used X-rays- radiation! An acid approach!! Acid destroys cells!

Conclusion

Boston had received 1 round of vaccinations (he was due His boosters) within a few weeks, his body had initiated sickness/vomiting. This is one of the body's natural flushing mechanisms; it is an innate response this amazing machine has. The anti-sickness and anti-bacterial injection has suppressed this natural ability along with also attacking the good bacteria (part of the immune system- which is still developing) this results in locking as well as pushing the toxicity (acidity) further into the body, the fever was generated by the body to burn what it had been prevented from attempting to remove, further steroids and synthetic foods were given, burdening the lymphatic system (body's sewer system) thus we witnessed swollen lymph nodes as it backs up creating constipation, the body still fighting yet being prevented from protecting itself (its cells) a number of further fevers are witnessed and prevented thus we see the toxicity and added toxicity pushed deeper into the body and into the joints, breaking down the mucus membrane! Means that the cells cannot function with ease, thus without true awareness of causation, a final diagnosis of 'Idiopathic poly arthritis' is given, a result of what has been consumed or what has been forced into the body on this occasion) cause and effect, disease (dis-ease of motion or function) does not come from anywhere.

Chapter 8: The Physical-Direct Approach To Assisting The Body In Healing

No matter what the disease (dis-ease of motion or function), the cause is always the same; thus, the approach should always be the same – cut out all causation and cleanse the body at a cellular level. The method should be as follows.

1. Fasting

Fasting, as I say, is "THE FOUNDATIONS OF HEALING", as mentioned Professor Ehret called it, the "MASTER KEY" Mr Hippocrates "THE FATHER OF MEDICINE" stated, *"to eat when you are sick, is to feed your sickness"* Dr Sebi used fasting to heal Himself and others too, fasting is naturally initiated by the body and is a natural phenomenon.

"How can we expect to cleanse the body on a cellular level as well as flush the lymphatic system if we continue to feed the system?"

2. Cleanse the Colon

Dr Sebi always stated that before any dis-ease can be reversed (with the cause removed), the colon must first be targeted; with your understanding of the lymphatic system as well as the body at a cellular level now, this should be easy to grok why!

3. Revitalise the cells to help maintain strength in the body.

With certain herbs, the body can be supported with energy and the blood kept clean as well as healthy. Again, this is easy to grasp, knowing the importance of blood flow, lymphatic drainage, and the fact the body is electrical.

4. Address the issue.

Upon cleansing the colon alongside helping to revitalise the cells (with minerals) as well as keeping them hydrated, the main issue can then be addressed, ensuring that the correct herbs and again approach is used, with the same inner standing that we are cleansing the body at a cellular level whilst at the same time revitalising the body.

At this stage, your thoughts might be somewhere along the lines of "herbs? I thought dogs were carnivores" I do stand firm in this understanding and for obvious reasons pointed out in this book, however It was stated in many scriptures that "The herbs are for the healing of the nations" with this in mind as well as going back to nature I would like to point out that all animals consume a SARF diet but alongside that and above food is water (around 70% of the body is water), water is processed by the body regardless of whether the animal is a carnivore, omnivore, herbivore or frugivore, so my advice to people is always to make herbal tonics, we use an acid approach (heating the herbs) pulling the natural benefits of the herb into the water molecule, the water is not only absorbed much quicker into the body (as its liquid) but we have infused the plant benefit, meaning that it will assimilate through the cell structure, essentially we are simply using these herbal tonics to help cleanse the body at a cellular level, however they can be used to restrengthen too as the minerals will assist in regeneration and cell strength.

This approach of fasting which really is dependent on the severity of the issue alongside the use of herbal tonics, is for a period of time whilst cleansing, helping to bring about the body's innate ability to regenerate itself (its cells) once we have established the cleansing along with bringing homeostasis back to the body, this approach can then be terminated, however, due to the fact we have an inner world to cleanse (around 75 trillion cells with two gigantic fluid based vessels) it's a big job, so faith, as well as patience, is always a factor, this can be demonstrated with many of our shop customers who have shared with us their journeys as not all have seen quick results, some results have taken months, but again results are based on the approach as well as the health issue we are dealing with.

Proven Method Used To Assist The Body In Healing

With almost all disease, and as you will now hopefully be aware of, the approach is to cleanse the body at a cellular level. This is accomplished with the use of herbal tonics alongside a fasting plan. The herbal tonics aim to cleanse through the cell, and specific herbs are required allowing us to address certain areas of the body. The following method is what I have successfully used a number of times for skin disease or skin-related issues due to toxicity created from constipation as a result of what has been allowed to enter the body. This approach has also been successful in reversing pancreatic issues and liver disease.

Colon Cleanse Kit

I use and recommend a mix of herbs that make up this cleansing tonic. This tonic is then given last thing on an evening at least 4 hours after feeding (please see below fasting guide). I would normally advise a colon cleanse for 3-4 weeks, sometimes longer, depending on the severity of constipation within the body.

Following on from the colon cleanse tonic, I also advise the use of slippery elm (powder). This can also be made into a tonic and is to be given the day after the colon cleanse is initiated at least 4 hrs after food or 1 hr again, before (please see below fasting guide). This again is to be given in line with the colon cleanse for 3-4 weeks and acts not only as a digestive tonic but also as a digestive lubricant assisting the body in the elimination of waste.

Blood, Liver, Skin, Gall bladder, Kidney and Lymph Cleanse

This mixture generally consists of several herbs all of which target the above areas of the body. The herbs can be switched and changed depending on the cause. This tonic is to be given 4 hrs after food or at least 1 hr before (please see below fasting guide). This will also be given in line with the colon cleanse for 3-4 weeks.

As most of these herbs are bitter – (alkalinity is bitter, acidity is sweet), more often than not either bone broths have to be given alongside them or I recommend using the blood that can be taken from the minces that are used regularly today when feeding a SARF diet and one I strongly advocate, if you still struggle getting your dog/s to consume the tonics a 5ml syringe can be used and although in some cases it can be difficult to get your dog to take the tonics, it has been shown time and time again that patience, perseverance and persistence makes way for a dog that not only gets used to the bitterness and begins accepting the bitter tonics but also is key to accomplishing the healing results desired, on the odd occasion that a dog doesn't take to the tonics, it should be noted that this method is only going to be for a short period in relation to their life span, its only to assist the body in cleansing, this said, the above method may also need to be initiated more than once, in some cases it has to be continued in order to cleanse what in reality is an inner world with around 75 trillion cells making up the body alongside a vast pipework network of venous (blood) and lymphatic (sewer system) vessels.

Before we look at the fasting protocol, I want to remind you of L.D. Mech and the fact that dogs are, by all scientific standards and evolutionary history, a direct descendant of the grey wolf, it has been L.D. Mechs observations that wolves can go up to six weeks without eating when there is no food available. When we also remember that there are no set meals, set times or set amounts in nature and that most animals fast all the time, we can Grok that a 5-day fast as recommended below is, in fact, a drop in the ocean to what dogs are capable of, in fact, I have observed numerous customers dogs over the years fast themselves up to and beyond five days when they're attempting to get their own way with a particular food type or flavour, simply because they can.

Fasting protocol – standard build-up to 5 days fast to start at the same time as taking the herbal tonics.

1 day fast + plenty of fresh water + herbal tonics

2-day feeding + plenty of fresh water + herbal tonics (1 hr before and 4 hrs after food)

2-days fast + plenty of fresh water + herbal tonics

2-days feeding + plenty of fresh water + herbal tonics (1 hr before and 4 hrs after food)

3 days fast + plenty of fresh water + herbal tonics

2-day feeding + plenty of fresh water + herbal tonics (1 hr before and 4 hrs after food)

4 days fast + plenty of fresh water + herbal tonics

2-day feeding + plenty of fresh water + herbal tonics (1 hr before and 4 hrs after food)

5-day fast + plenty of fresh water + herbal tonics

Following are some of the visual results I have witnessed and experienced as part of using this method. I would like to point out that the more severe issues and states of disease seen below are with dogs that have been prescribed Apoquel

as a systematic approach to what had started as an allergy! –
which I discussed earlier in the book.

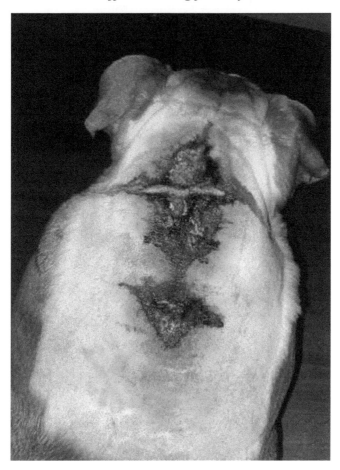

At this stage, The Vet didn't know the cause, or in fact, that their approach had created this condition. The decision at this point was going to be to end Jaffa's life. You can read Jaffa's owners' personal journey below

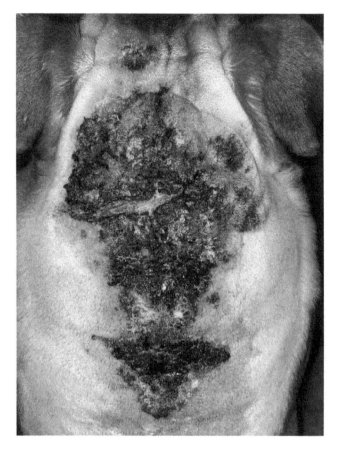

This was a few days into the cleansing and fasting method. You can see we now have a wound that is beginning to heal as it begins to scab over.

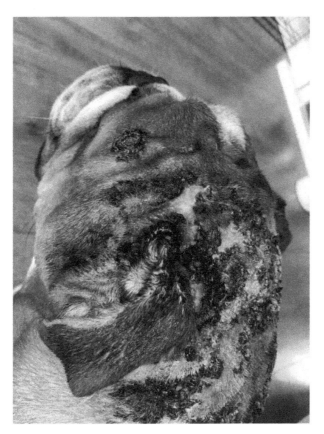

At this stage, Jaffa's body had begun to eliminate the toxicity and the toxicity release spread creating the appearance of the wound spreading up to his head. The below image shows how much of Jaffa's body was affected by the cleanse due to the level of toxicity.

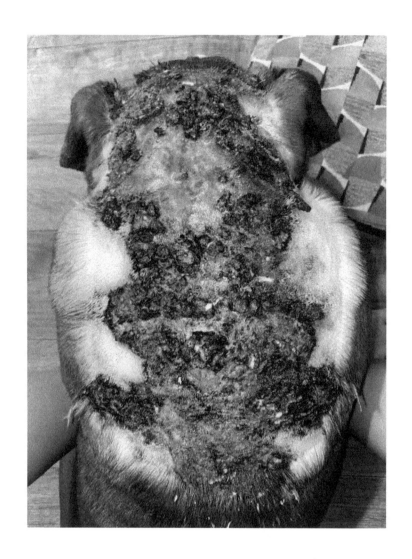

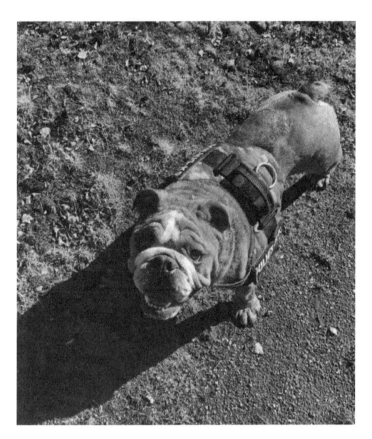

This was just six weeks after Jaffa began his Herbal tonics and fasting protocol. 75% of the damage that had been created (constipation/parasites) had been dealt with, and Jaffa's body had regenerated because we removed the cause. Jaffa's journey was one of the worst visually, but quickest recoveries I have witnessed to date.

Jaffa's owner's journey

"Here is my English bulldog Jaffa. Three years of age. Always been fit, healthy, strong, and have the clearest airways, usually went on walks up to around 8 miles. Around the 9th of July we noticed a funky smell and puss coming from Jaffa's back. We thought maybe this was a hotspot. He

had a hotspot before, but very small. We took Jaffa to the vet, and was instantly put on antibiotics. Jaffa was already on long-term steroids for ten months prior to this appointment for chronic ear infections. They also upped his steroids to try and stop the "hotspot" from spreading. Long story short, it did not stop. It spread so quickly, and after a vet appointment every two days of us worrying, they didn't know what it was and kept giving Jaffa more antibiotics and upping his steroids. They gave us creams, washes, and different tablets including Apoquel. Nothing stopped this disease from eating away at his body. It smelt, it was wet, it was raw and extremely painful for him. We decided to go to a dermatologist instead as we got nowhere at this point, and this infection had spread from palm size to covering the majority of his back. She took some blood, skin scrapes and then prescribed further antibiotics and washes. We stuck with it again but started to see a drastic change in Jaffa. He had no energy, lethargic, couldn't stand, couldn't walk, couldn't lift his head up, eyes rolling to the back of his head, and 10+ head tremors a day. Jaffa cried all the time; he would try and smash his head into the walls when the head tremors started to make it stop and would make himself bleed from biting or scratching against surfaces. He was in such an ill state. The dermatologist advised us at that point it would be a "fair" decision to put Jaffa down because he wasn't responding to treatment, and they said further tests would take months and months, but Jaffa probably wouldn't make it. We had exhausted everything we thought we could. Spent thousands of pounds at this point and didn't know what disease was eating away at our little boy's skin. We were one day away from putting Jaffa down... by some miracle, a man went into my mum's salon and recommended coming here urgently before taking Jaffa to the vets. We weren't too sure anything would work at that point. We were all exhausted, and I was heartbroken for Jaffa going through so much pain every day. But I and my partner had to try everything before giving up. And boy, am I glad we did. Gareth is incredible at what he does, and his knowledge is second to none. He spoke to us in-depth and explained why Jaffa's body wasn't healing. He immediately said, "I'm confident Jaffa's still got life in him, and we can turn this around." And he was absolutely right. We took Jaffa off every single medication he was on the same day. We started a detox. Fasting him gradually up to a five day fast. He was on a herbal tea that I made, recommended by Gareth, 3x a day. We have done this for the last six weeks. And let me tell you. Jaffa was not able to walk, stand up for longer than 2 minutes or lift his head off the sofa for the last three months, until now. He's better than ever before, running around, happy every day, sleeping on his back because he's now able to get comfortable; he's playing, jumping. It's honestly the best feeling in the world, knowing he's happy and feeling well again. I know Gareth will say it's been a team effort but hand on my heart, I cannot thank this man enough for *essentially saving our Jaffa. Thank you so much. I cannot recommend him enough. This was caused by a build-up of toxins, medications, steroids, antibiotics, things his body did not need! His body was close to giving up when all it was screaming for was to stop having the meds from the vets and to allow his body to heal with natural remedies. Before anyone allows their pet to get to this stage, please just see this man and get some advice! He truly knows his stuff. THANK YOU!"*

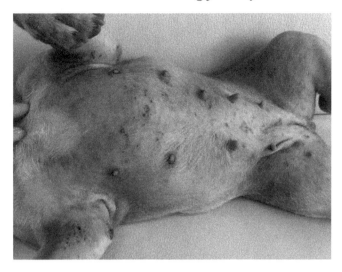

Nala had also been on meds to treat "allergies." Her skin is burdened as Her body pushes out toxicity. Luckily for Nala, her owners came to me early on, and she didn't undergo years of immune-suppressing meds.

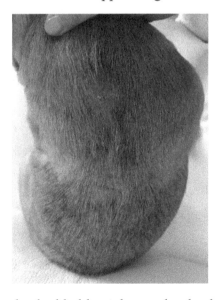

Nala also had bald patches on her back too.

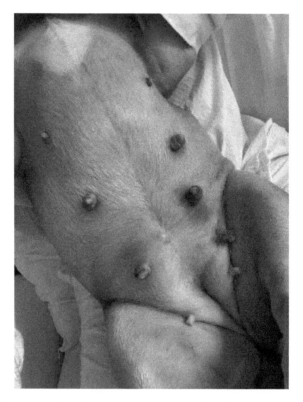

This was after just over one month of cleansing Nala's body at a cellular level. The following photo also shows her back healthy too.

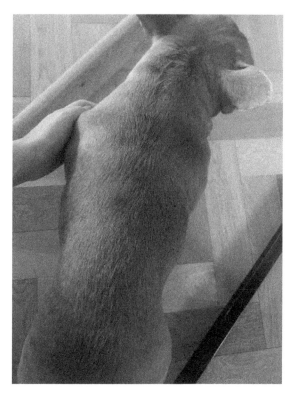

Nala's Owners Journey

"Here are our before and after photos of our 1.5-year-old Frenchie.

We have followed Gareth's advice and have been giving her herbal teas, raw food and fasting her; we also came off of steroids and anti-allergy tablets all since the middle of August.

We first completed the FULL fast program that Gareth recommended to us with the herbal teas, which took around a month. We had no days off; we completed the whole thing without any breaks and no missed teas; we were on it!

(Yes, I felt awful for her, however, I want her to get better, so sometimes you have to be cruel to be kind).

For this week, you've told us to try a different tea, so we've dropped the other three teas and will run this one and see how she goes.

It's only been a couple of months, but my god, you can see a difference. We still have a way to go, but I'm so happy with her results so far.

Thank you so much for your help, we really appreciate it!

Alicia"

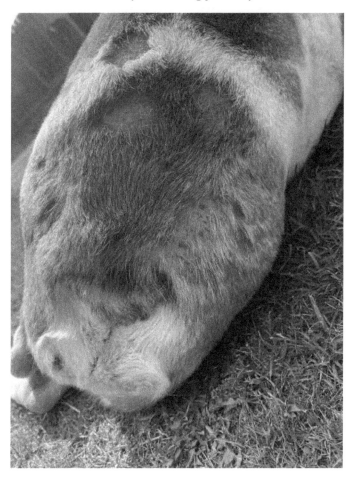

Buddy's owner initially came to us for advice to get his weight down due to a luxating patella issue and was seeking to switch to a SARF diet after a recommendation from a customer. I always like to get the history of the dog and its back ground to get a feel for potentially how toxic the body is internally; this is what Buddy looked like initially, eight months before we started the cleanse.

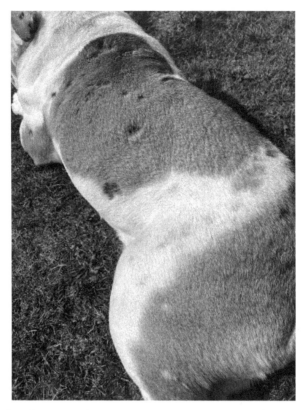

Further images show the bald patches on Buddy's body
where the skin is being used to filter out toxicity.

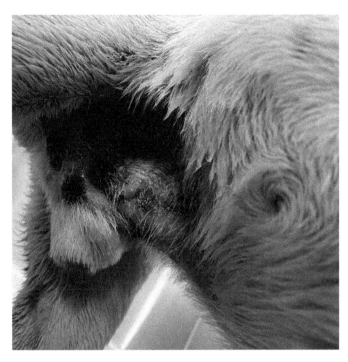

This picture of Buddy is a month or so into the cleanse; what we tend to see with cleansing is a worsening of the issue as the body begins to eliminate the inflammation/toxicity via the largest eliminative organ filter, the skin. It also identifies that His Kidneys are struggling hence the skin is being used more so now to filter as we assist the body in cleansing the root of His issue. Notice how aggressive the cleanse is and what was, up until now, being prevented from elimination and stored in the body as opposed to allowing the body to remove it.

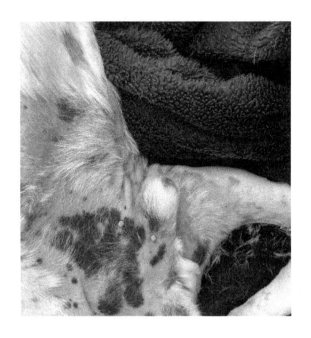

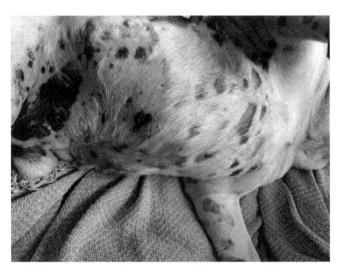

The above two images are from a few weeks after. We can see the skin calming down now as the majority of the inflammation/toxicity has been allowed to be removed. It also shows how much fur had been lost in the cleanse.

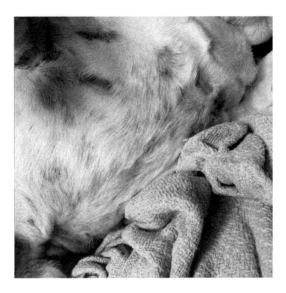

The above images show us we're in the regeneration process and Buddy's body has removed the majority of toxicity. We can clearly see the skin is now much healthier and a natural pink colour, and Buddy's fur has also started growing back.

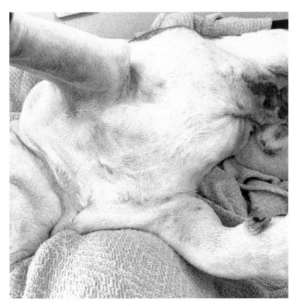

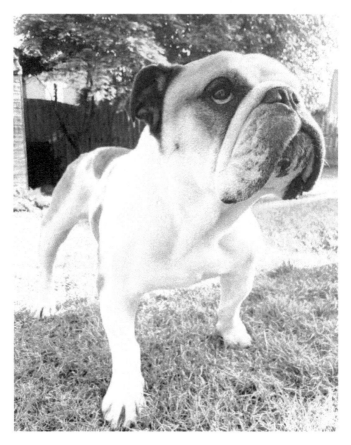

This is where we are today with Buddy. As you can see now, Buddy has a full new coat (the body regenerates itself when we remove causation) and now looks and feels so much softer, as well as being much healthier because the cells are functioning with ease.

Buddy's Owners Journey

"Our Boy Buddy has been on a full cleanse as recommended. He was on Apoquel from the vets for a long time to manage allergies but didn't really correct the issues. He then suddenly started limping on one of his back legs.

I was so panicked; I took him to the Vet straight away, who said his knee was popping in and out as he walked and would be in pain.

I was advised to put him on rheumocam for the pain. This then eased it.

They did tell me he would need surgery for this and that it wouldn't heal, I was at my wit's end as he's not insured as it was too costly for me at the time, plus at this time, he was fine anyway. To Help Buddy with this knee issue, I then decided to take Him for hydrotherapy and decided on Aquapaws Canine Hydrotherapy & Fun Swim Barnsley and try to get his weight down to stop him from limping as much.

I had been taking Buddy to hydro for a couple of weeks, but he was putting on weight which didn't make sense to me at first, but then I realised, it was because of the muscle mass He was building around the joint, I had talked about Buddy's issues to the team at Aquapaws who advised that I might be better speaking with sure4pets to see if they can help me with what he's eating as I was cutting down on what he had anyways.

Gareth Sheppard talked me through the whole back-to-nature way, going right back to basics! It was a lot of info, and I still have to ask questions every now and again, but I'm so, So glad that I found this place to help me through all of this as for me surgery was not an option I wanted to take.

So, at this moment in time, Buddy is on a 2-day feed then he will be three days fasting with his herbal teas!

He's really sore at the minute but Gareth assured me again that this is all normal and it will get worse before it's better.

He's also given me a natural recipe to be used as an anti-inflammatory! I can't wait to see more results with these herbal teas! They have saved our boy from becoming an absolute mess full of toxins. "NEVER AGAIN!" will I give him anything other than what comes from the ground!

I'm so happy I could cry! The hard work and determination from myself and Sure4Pets have finally paid off! And he's on the up from now on!

So originally, I went to the vet with my buddy because he was limping. He said he would need surgery, He was then given pain relief medication to keep him comfortable so I could save for the surgery and x-ray....

I then asked sure4pets Limited to see what I could do to help him lose a bit of weight, as this wasn't helping his knee issue. He then told me about fasting and herbal teas to help him lose more weight and to help repair his cells that are damaged!

It all started back in April, so in 8 months, we've had these herbal teas and fasting & he's doing so well with it. He absolutely hates the tea's lol, and I do have to syringe it in his mouth for him to have it.... It's literally like having a second child, but I love Him, so I'll keep doing it till he's 100%

He's now not on any pain medication or anything else from the vets, and he's doing amazing!

So the last pictures are from September last year & the first pictures are of BUDDY today, 30-5-2023

He's done so well; bless him!

Come such a long way, and he's so lean now!

With help from Gareth Sheppard - AKA -Alpha Canine Health and the team at sure4pets Limited, he's a brand new dog!

Still keeping up with the herbal teas and fasting on odd occasions, but he's brand new! His skin is on tip-top condition now compared to before! "

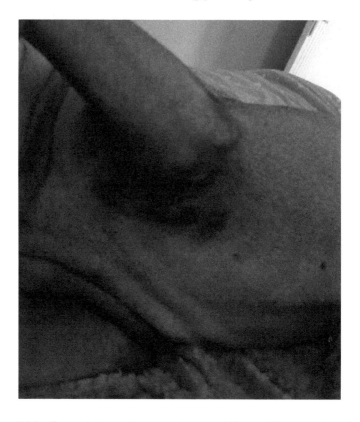

This first picture shows the condition of Rolo when his owner first came to the shop. He was fed a commercial–synthetic diet, regular flea, worm and vaccination treatments. I initiated a fast along with a cleansing protocol.

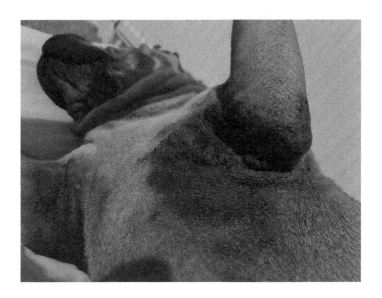

As you will see from this photo and after only two weeks of fasting and a specific herbal compound approach, the disease worsened as Rolo's body began to remove the cause, and as you can imagine, at this stage, the owner became extremely concerned, I assured him this does tend to happen, and he persevered with the protocol and kept his faith in the process.

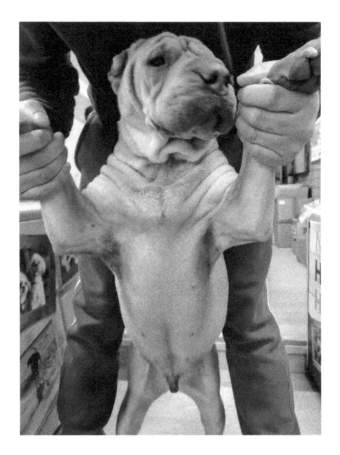

This is Rolo 10 months after we initiated the cleansing protocol. It took faith, patience and perseverance from Rolo's owner to get Rolo back to health with the natural approach used, and these are the results. As you can imagine, Rolo's owner is very happy with the results and glad He persisted even when He had doubts.

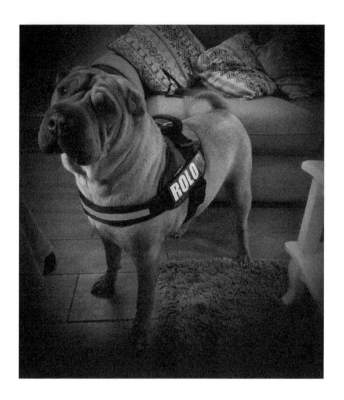

Rolo's Owners Journey

"After taking the shop's advice, we fasted Rolo (and have continued this for two days a week). We have changed his diet to a variety of raw meats - previously. He just had lamb. We have been giving him tonics and sea moss as advised. He has always had issues with his skin underneath, his feet and ears etc. Since starting this, his skin has been much worse, it now looks painful, and for the first time, he is scratching it.

The first photo was Rolo's skin when we first visited the shop and took advice from Gareth.

2nd photo was taken a few weeks later after fasting, using herbal teas and a fully raw diet. It was getting worse before it got better.

His skin was extremely sore, cracked and causing him to scratch until he was bleeding. We were going to stop when it got this bad as it was awful to see, but Gareth advised us to persevere, and advised that it would clear up.

It has taken ten months, but as you can see from the 3rd photo, his skin is nearly clear.

100% recommend."

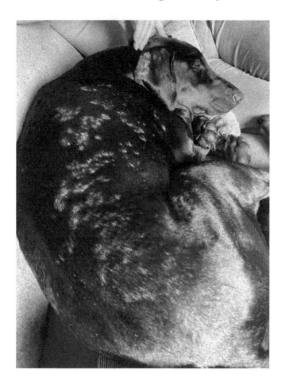

This was Luna's skin and coat condition when Her owner first came to us; her owner had exhausted all the mainstream approaches and was reluctant to accept that Steroids would be the only means to manage the condition.

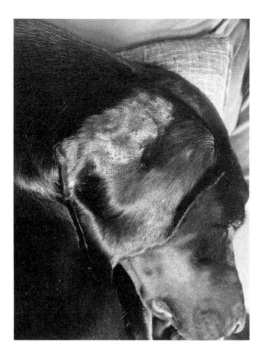

Again this headshot shows the condition of Luna's skin at this point.

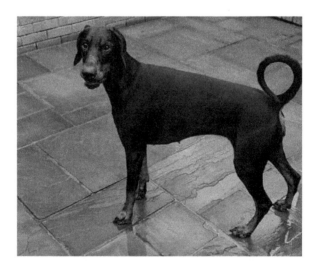

This image is just 17 days after Luna started her fast and herbal cleanse. As you can see, her skin has already cleared up, and her fur has not only grown back but is now shining just as it should be.

Luna's Owners Journey

"Long post! From about 8 months old, Luna developed a skin condition. I tried everything biopsy, blood tests, changing diet, a million and one different shampoos and skin products, but nothing seemed to make any difference. In the end, Luna got diagnosed with perivascular dermatitis, and I was told If this didn't clear the only thing they could do for her was to take steroids.

With her being only 20 months old, this was not an option. I continued to look for more natural ways around this problem, often getting demoralised and frustrated and feeling hopeless for her. But in the end, I found sure4pets a shop local to me and Gareth, who said that he had dealt with things like this and had roughly an 80% success rate. But the diet seemed scary to understand and get my head around. I felt bad and even called the lady who bred her and spoke with her about it, who reassured me that I knew my dog, and that I will make the right decision for her. It's a herb and root fasting diet. (Fasting allows the body to focus purely on recovery) we start a fast at 36 hrs and feed for two days, then increase the fast by 12 hours and feed for two days. We are currently on the final fast of 5 days. During the fast, she will have bone broth and herbal tea from the herbs/roots to fill her body with minerals and cleanse her body of the toxins being released from the skin, causing the dry skin/rashes three times a day. The pictures show how bad her skin was. The last photo is just from 17 days of this diet! Please, if you have lost all hope of fixing your dog's bad skin, I cannot recommend this process enough. I finally have my dog back, and she's back to herself. I have my tactical donkey back. Your advice and help means so much more than you will ever know or realise, and for anyone worried like I was about the fasting, Luna has lost next to no weight at all. She's still super active, wanting to play, and hasn't changed in the slightest apart from her skin getting better day by day. Again, thank you so, so much Gareth – AlphaCanineHealth."

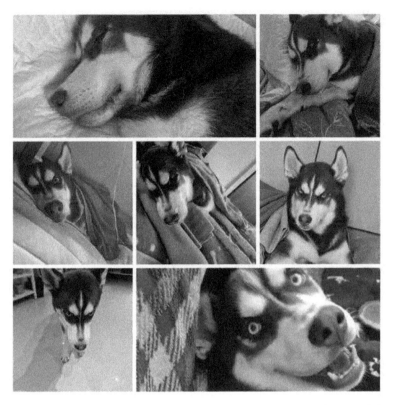

Although there doesn't seem much to observe here with Coba's condition, and the images certainly don't do the severity of the problem justice, He was in a critical condition and the vets didn't hold much hope for him. Coba's body had already initiated a fast, meaning that all I had to do was support Him further with a compound of herbs that allowed us to neutralise the cause which was in the intestines. For a dog that wasn't expected to see the night out, He made a superb recovery and is once again loving life.

Coba's Owners Journey

"This is my beautiful puppy, Coba. Last week he was diagnosed with a parvo virus, and he was given a 10 % chance of surviving the night. The vet was CONVINCED He would not make it and kept telling me that my puppy would die and that I wouldn't be able to do anything to save him. I rang Gareth on the recommendation of a friend and asked him for help. He was supportive from the first minute! He used all his knowledge, and what's most important, he put his heart into saving Coba. With Gareth, my puppy was given a 100 % chance for the best and longest life. He supported me in every single step, and even gave him the first dose of herbs! In my whole life, I have never felt so grateful to anyone as I'm now with Gareth. He is the best that could have happened to my puppy and me. The pictures showed Coba from last week when he was diagnosed with parvo virus and now. In only 6 days from diagnosis, my Coba has started to eat on his own, drink water, walk, play, and bark. The road to the full recovery is still long, but I'm more than confident that everything will be ok. The vaccination and vet don't guarantee anything, and Coba is a great example of this! I could not recommend Gareth and Sure4pets more!!!!"

These examples are just some of the successful healing journeys that I have assisted people's dogs with; most issues I have seen tend to be with skin, which is simply a filter and, as already mentioned, is part of the immune system – skin, blood, and lymph, these symptoms are simply a fault code from the body and require our understanding of the body in order to be able to assist the body in removing what is causing the disease – dis-ease of function or motion within this system and wherever that might be. The approach I use is what I call the Canine Bio-mineral Balance ™ under this approach, I use an intra-cellular cleanse and intra-cellular revitalisation ™ providing cell food ™ with a selection of herbs that come under the approach that I call the Canine Bio-mineral Balance ™ assisting the body in removing the cause of the problem through a cleansing process which uses organic (electric) herbs that allow cell assimilation, meaning that it will cleanse through the cell, thus providing a superior result long term, however long that might be because as you will also find from the above examples, there are no rules to healing, some are seen quickly, and others take time, but one thing is for sure and as I always reaffirm to people – 'understanding, patience, persistence and above all faith in nature and the Canine Bio-mineral Balance ™ process of healing is key.'

Conclusion

We have covered what I see currently as the main areas that are critical in ensuring health in life for our canine companions who, over the past 150 years, have seen a huge decline in life spans and their health between. I have provided you with what I hope to be a concise as well as a basic explanation with the direction of the actions required to help ensure that we can provide the health, vitality, and life longevity these animals, along with all animals, deserve, I trust that you are now able to Grok the cause of disease, how we can assist the body in dealing with the disease naturally, but more importantly the prevention of disease, I'm hoping that you will also discern that unnecessary work (digestion of none Species Appropriate Raw Foods will tax the body (it takes energy to digest food) thus we are wearing it down unnecessarily as well as in many cases knocking the body out of homeostasis (its chemical balance), Let's get the life spans back up to what they should be and what they deserve!.

Science Definition

The intellectual and practical activity encompasses the systematic study of the structure and behaviour of the physical and natural world through observation and experiment.

Does this definition imply that its only subject to a group of people within a socially structured system or that to use, apply and have the presented science accepted, you must have a degree from the system?

How can humanity truly progress if we limit ourselves only to what is told by people that are "trained or credentialed" that simply parrot the current status quo -IE government backed narrative within the programmed system, IE Vets, Dr's, Media, etc. that are not willing to look at other research and in many cases ignores past science unless it fits their portrayal, it clearly identifies the ignorance that exists in this system, meaning that it doesn't denote that they are better informed but are blinding themselves and others by ignoring what doesn't fit their narrative, which is simply programming!.

References

Wayne, R.K. "What is a Wolfdog?"
(www.fiu.edu/~milesk/Genetics.html), (Feldhamer, G.A.
1999. Mammology: Adaptation, Diversity, and Ecology.
McGraw-Hill.

(Wayne, R.K. Molecular Evolution of the Dog Family).
Mech, L.D.

(Ronald Schultz)

Billinghurst, n.d

Dr Ronald Schultz, Dr Jeannie Thomason, Dr Robert
Morse, Dr Patricia Jordan, Dr Edward. Shook, L.
David.Mech, Dr Ian Billingshurst, Robert.K. Wayne,
Lonsdale, Brown & Taylor, Pottinger, Professor Arnold
Ehret, Dr Joe Dispenza, Hippocrates, Dr Sebi